Wabi Sabi

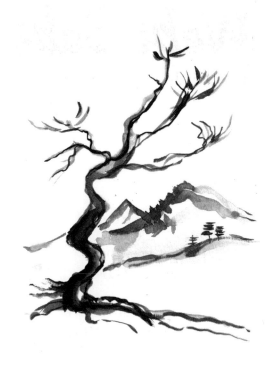

Wabi Sabi

The Wisdom in Imperfection

Nobuo Suzuki

Foreword by
Héctor García

Translated from Spanish by
Russell Andrew Calvert

TUTTLE Publishing

Tokyo | Rutland, Vermont | Singapore

CONTENTS

*"The straight line belongs to men,
the curved one to God."*

—ANTONI GAUDÍ

Foreword

I remember clearly the first time I heard the term *wabi sabi*. It was fifteen years ago on a live TV show in Japan. I was really nervous at the start of the interview but I found that I could follow the questions and answer in my beginner level Japanese. Until the announcer said: "What do you think about wabi sabi?"

I had no idea what wabi sabi is, and I was on live TV! I couldn't just whip out my phone and look it up. After a brief, awkward pause, I answered with something totally unrelated. It was obvious that I didn't understand the question.

The shame I felt from that experience set me on an adventure of studying and learning about wabi sabi and Japanese aesthetics in general, an adventure that continues to this day. Most certainly, wabi sabi is one of the greatest things I've learned from the Japanese people, and it's had a powerful effect on who I am as a person and on my world view.

I asked all my Japanese friends, my coworkers, my girlfriend, all the new people I met: What is wabi sabi? What do you think about wabi sabi? What is wabi sabi for you? After a while I realized that no two answers would ever be the same, but all of them had a common essence: life and the universe we live in is all about the imperfection and impermanence of all things.

I soon came to realize that wabi sabi is more than aesthetics. It's about life, being human and even about the universe in general. It's about the ephemeral nature of all things and learning to accept that, even to embrace it. Wabi sabi is an invisible texture that interconnects Japanese art, lifestyle, architecture, history, philosophy, religions and even Japanese thought, social behavior and mindset.

Western thought, and more specifically, modernity, pushes all of us to think that there is an ultimate perfect goal in all things we do that will lead us to success and happiness. Nobuo Suzuki helps us to reflect deeply on this supposed aim to success, and on how we live in modern cities. His words helped me to remember that perfection does not even exist to begin with; it is only in the realm of our human imagination (and mathematics, maybe).

Wabi sabi is reality.

Perfection does not exist.

After being bathed in the wisdom of wabi sabi I started experiencing Japan through different eyes. I noticed that I'd begun to look at Japanese bowls with fascination instead of indifference, the way my younger self did. I also started enjoying and admiring its gardens, poetry, pottery, ikebana and architecture more.

The change in my thinking and perception wasn't limited to how I see Japan and things Japanese. When I was traveling back through Europe I noticed that I had a renewed interest in all types of art, but also in people—in different lifestyles, and in my family and friends in all of their wonderful imperfections. Everything had new value for me.

In retrospect I realized something funny: I didn't have to feel ashamed of my answer on TV—because wabi sabi can't really be explained, my answer was probably "correct." Moreover, it's ok to be imperfect, it's ok to not know something (even when asked on television).

Wabi Sabi: the Wisdom in Imperfection is a beautiful exploration that goes from the basics of wabi sabi to its deeper meaning in all its facets. This book does not pretend to offer a definitive explanation of the wabi sabi philosophy, but it will make you want to dive into the concept, and so change forever the way you think and feel about yourself and the world we all share.

After reading this book, I've found myself more aware of wabi sabi everywhere in my day-to-day– while working and interacting with others, when I'm walking in nature or in a city, and when I am doing nothing in particular. I'm also more aware of the pain we put ourselves through when we live at odds with wabi sabi, constantly trying to perfect our lives, to climb "higher," to get "better" jobs, "better" houses, "better" routines and "better" everything. In today's world, we are infected with thoughts like "I missed the chance to accomplish this or that," "I'm not achieving enough," "I will never be as good as…," and in this way we talk ourselves into feeling inadequate and unworthy. And we shouldn't. We are beautiful beings whose goals and expectations have been misshaped by modern values. Why are we all aiming to have a perfect life that does not even exist?

Wabi sabi is about learning to be ok with whatever it is that we are and with what we have in this moment. It doesn't take away our responsibility to strive to be better, more fully alive people. It means that once we realize that we are ok with the present moment, we move ahead every day, step by step, aiming not toward perfection, but toward our best selves—to discover the essence of who we really are, our *ikigai*. This idea of freeing ourselves of unrealistic expectations in order to move forward, to become better, is one of the many lovely takeaways you'll find in the pages of this book.

Certainly, I know more now about wabi sabi than I did when I first heard the term fifteen years ago. But I can also say that the more I know about wabi sabi, the deeper it runs in me, and I will never get tired of it.

This book has taken me to some new places on my journey through wabi sabi. Its perspective refreshes my enthusiasm for the experience of being alive in the world as it is. And, it's helped me to appreciate the wabi sabi philosophy even more and to cherish it as a guide on how to live my life.

Let's embrace our imperfect selves and our imperfect world, to see that world's beauty and thereby make it even more beautiful. Nobuo Suzuki's book can start you on that path. I hope you'll enjoy reading it as much as I did.

—Héctor García
Tokyo, October 2020

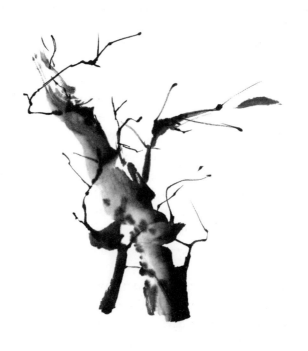

PROLOGUE
The Magic of Imperfection

It is said there was a monk in charge of the garden of a Zen monastery in Japan who had a peculiar habit. When sweeping the fall leaves from the stone path, he would let one leaf fall to the ground just before going back inside his house.

Why did he do that?

For one thing, the trees themselves would soon sprinkle the path with more golden leaves. For another, the Japanese ideal of beauty does not seek perfection, uniformity and exact symmetry, but naturalness: the beauty conveyed by a fallen leaf in the empty garden of a Zen monastery.

One of the distinguishing features of Japanese culture is its peculiar concept of beauty. For a Westerner, even for a Chinese, the most beautiful cup is an impeccably fashioned one, with a perfect circumference, a smooth immaculate surface and—if it is decorated—an exact and uniform arrangement of the decorations.

In Japan, however, the most highly-prized cup—and the most expensive—tends to be the one that contains flaws, because that makes it unique. It may have dents, sandstone stuck to it or even be cracked or mended through the art of *kintsugi*, which we shall talk about later on in this book.

As well as being unique and telling its own tale, this oh-so-special cup transmits the Japanese spirit of *wabi sabi*, which regards things that resemble nature as beautiful, and which may be summed up with the following three principles:

1. Nothing is perfect
2. Nothing is finished.
3. Nothing lasts forever.

Applied to humans, being aware of our imperfection makes us humble; accepting it frees us from being unhealthily self-demanding and from the fixation on a perfection that does not exist in nature and by extension does not exist in humans either.

Accepting our own imperfection and each person's unique nature does not mean resignation. On the contrary, it shows us the path to follow to evolve as human beings.

Anyone who believes they have achieved excellence is both wrong—there is always room for improvement—and lacking in flexibility. Secure in their absolute and subjective truth, they have no margin for growth. Such a person is rigid and fossilized and does not exude life.

Moving on to the second principle, wabi sabi reminds us precisely that nothing is finished. Just as nature develops infinitely, amid cycles of births and deaths, so too are humans dynamic.

The Buddha himself once said: *"I am always beginning."*

Taking a wabi sabi approach to life means, once you have recognized your own imperfection, embracing continuous learning and assuming that *everything is still to be done*, and therefore, that *everything is still to be lived*.

The third principle of wabi sabi is understanding the fleeting nature of all that exists, a concept that takes us back to Zen. To come back to the Buddha once again, he pointed out, when talking about suffering, that one of its causes is that humans wish that things that by nature are transitory are permanent.

Youth flies and becomes maturity and then old age.

That fantastic television you have just bought eventually stops working or becomes outdated or obsolete. That person who seemed so charming and amusing stops surprising us, or maybe we start to drift apart because, like two branches of a tree, we have grown in opposite directions.

Rather than saddening us, accepting that *nothing lasts forever* inspires us to value the beauty of the moment, which is the only thing we can capture here and now. It is an invitation to give our everything to whatever we may be doing.

It might be the last time we go for a walk in the park but if we treat it as though we are saying farewell to life, it is worth all the walks in the world.

For the Japanese concept of beauty, in the same way that the imperfect or repaired cup is the most valuable, the dry leaf about to fall from a bare branch is more moving than a lush flower-filled meadow.

That is the magic of wabi sabi, which inspires our life offering us a new horizon of sensitivity, growth and self-fulfillment.

—NOBUO SUZUKI

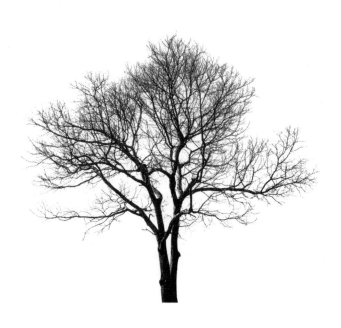

A MEDITATION

The cawing of the crows,
the snow-covered tōrō that looks like a bokushi in a hat,
the weight of the snow bending the tree branches,
the water from the fountain threading its way through the snow,
the sound of my footsteps deadened by the snow,
am I a tiny part of this imperfect garden?
or is the garden part of me, of my universe?

tōrō: a stone turret
bokushi: a monk

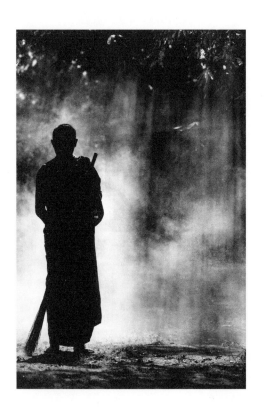

The Three Dimensions of Wabi Sabi

"From the temple in the mountain,
the sound of a bell strikes hesitantly,
disappears in the mist."
—Yosano Buson

For some time I have lived in a village where we all know one another. I begin my day walking from one end of the village to the other. I bow to the children going to school, to neighbors I have known for decades, to old people taking their dog out.

Each person goes where their *ikigai*—their reason for being—calls them. Some raise their hand in greeting, others bow or smile.

When I reach the southern end of the village, I pass the crimson-colored bridge as I enjoy the freshness of the river. I then feel the mountain air cleaning both my lungs and my thoughts. The murmur of the water tumbling over the rocks mixes sweetly with the tweeting of birds. I turn my head to take in the different green and orange hues of fall, encapsulated by the changing canvas of the tree canopy covering the mountains.

I pass through the wooden entrance to the temple and greet the monks who are sweeping the maple leaves that tumble down in late fall. Then I turn around and go home to my cat Tama to write.

All told, it is a walk of no more than forty-five minutes, but this time is crucial for my happiness.

Yesterday my friend Yūji came to visit. He is the editor of a literary magazine in Tokyo. I invited him to stroll with me and then we had tea in my living room, which looks out over the mountains.

"The smell of the tatami mixed with the scent of this green tea makes me nostalgic for my childhood," my friend said.

"It's an everyday aroma for me," I replied.

After a few minutes of shared silence while we enjoyed the Uji tea, good old Yūji said energetically:

"Nobuo… you should come to live in Tokyo. A man like you would be a success in the city."

"Be a success… and what is the good of that?"

"You'd be famous in literary circles and they'd invite you to events every day. You'd meet beautiful women there, influential people from the scene and you'd earn a lot of money. You'd have ten times as many professional opportunities as you have here, holed up in the mountains."

"Yeah… but with the stress of city life, I'd have ten times less inspiration. And ten times less happiness as well."

"Please, Nobuo," my friend begged me, "Don't be negative."

"Go to live in the city—why? To have more things I don't need?

"You're so Zen… You'll never change."

"Why accrue more than I need? I want to live true to my nature—wabi sabi is my guide."

"Wabi sabi is merely an aesthetic value," Yūji said. "It will help you with your art but with little else."

"For me, wabi sabi transcends all that," I protested. "It's a

22

philosophy and a way of life. I'd even go so far as to say it's a way of understanding the universe."

"That's all well and good but… aren't you afraid of making a mistake, of later regretting not having done anything apart from writing, playing the piano and walking in the mountains?"

I could not help but laugh at this question and exclaimed:

"The point is that in a wabi sabi life there *are* no mistakes. Life is imperfect by definition, so if I make a mistake, so be it!"

When my editor friend had gone, and while I contemplated the twilight with the cat on my lap, I thought that for me wabi sabi has three great dimensions.

Before stating what they are, I want to say that wabi sabi is with me from the moment I wake up until the time I go to bed. It is in the art I create and enjoy, it is in my house and garden, and also in my relationships with my family and friends. It is even in my relationship with my cat.

Wabi sabi is my way of feeling my existence and of interacting with the world elegantly, harmoniously and peacefully.

Yūji's visit inspired me to write this book, which will be divided into three main sections corresponding to the following dimensions:

I. WABI SABI PHILOSOPHY

In this first part, I will talk about wabi sabi as a worldview and existential philosophy. It gives us a different way of understanding and feeling both the universe and our relationships with others. Observing the world through the prism of wabi sabi will help you to live in harmony, both in times of peace and in times of stress and angst.

Wabi sabi philosophy tells us that everything is *impermanent*. Even rocks that have been forming a mountain for millions of years will one day disappear.

Everything is in a continual state of flux and if we go against the flow, we will suffer. The only way to be happy is to accept it. Sometimes we will feel melancholy and nostalgia, but these are feelings we can enjoy.

Why should we worry about the future or the present if nothing will be the same tomorrow as it was yesterday?

II. WABI SABI ART

As an aesthetic, more than allowing us to study works of art in more depth, understanding this concept lets us explore the soul of the objects surrounding us or the soul of our own home. Three examples of wabi sabi art:

- A traditional Japanese house whose structure has been restored while keeping the cracks in the hundred-year-old wood.
- A teacup that fell to the floor and broke into pieces but has been restored using *kintsugi* techniques.
- A movie in which the main theme is the imperfection of the characters and the passing of time in their lives. My countryman Yasujirō Ozu's movies are essentially wabi sabi.

III. WABI SABI AS A WAY OF LIFE

It is not enough to understand and feel wabi sabi if we do not live by its principles. In this third section, we shall see ideas for introducing this philosophy into daily life and improving it, with proposals such as:

- Continuing to use old objects but looking after them like old friends.
- Learning to say "no" to social or business propositions which may not be quite the opportunities they appear to be.
- Avoiding getting frustrated by life's imperfections, because no human being has a perfect life.
- Taking things as they are, accommodating twists in fate and making the best out of change in a life in which you are in harmony with yourself and with all that surrounds you, including your friends and family.
- Living in tune with nature: going for walks in the countryside or looking after plants in your garden or on your veranda.
- Practicing some kind of art which allows you to follow the aesthetic principles of wabi sabi.

With these three dimensions on the horizon, we are ready to begin a transformational journey toward the true nature of life and reality.

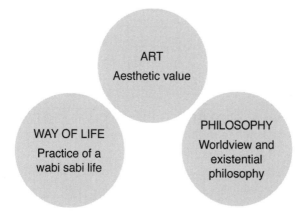

I

The Philosophy
of Wabi Sabi

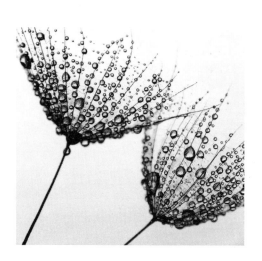

A MEDITATION

Perfection does not exist in the real world,
it merely dwells in the mind of human beings.
Not even the kami are perfect,
and nor do they aim to be so.
If the kami are not perfect,
nor wish to be so,
why do we humans aspire to perfection?

kami 神: a Japanese term used to refer to deities or spirits

Origins of the Concept

*"Pare down to the essence,
but don't remove the poetry."*
—LEONARD KOREN

Wabi sabi is a difficult expression to translate. Defining it precisely is not possible and would in any case show a lack of respect for my language. We Japanese like the ambiguity of our language and of life in general.

Ambiguity is beautiful because it always leaves the door open to possibilities.

The aim of this book is to explain, as far as possible, what the Japanese experience as wabi sabi in their daily life, without pigeonholing it with a specific definition.

If we stick to language, the expression is made up of the terms *wabi* and *sabi*. These two words may be used independently but almost always go together, as though a magnet wished them never to be separated.

The joining of the two can only be understood through history.

Evolution of the two terms
Oddly enough, both words started out with a negative emotional connotation, which has disappeared with the passing of the centuries. Personally, rather than making me feel sad,

going over these origins makes me feel nostalgic.

In the fourteenth century, when modern Japanese was still being formed, the word *wabi* began to be used by monks who followed the Zen tradition, going off to live alone in natural surroundings. These hermits used the word *wabi* to express the solitude one feels when living unaccompanied in nature.

What does solitude taste like?
How many types of solitude are there?

They had other words with which to express the common feeling of loneliness, but for the specific type of solitude felt in nature, for example, when we are alone in a forest, they used the word *wabi*.

With the passing of time, the meaning of the term gradually transformed and today *wabi* expresses tranquility, rustic simplicity and beautiful imperfections.

The second word that makes up this concept also emerged from the Zen Buddhism milieu. Previously, *sabi* had a meaning that was anything but positive. It was used to describe what is wizened, rotten, wilted or damaged. Just as with *wabi*, over time its meaning took on a positive connotation, and today *sabi* means the beauty and calm brought to us by a certain age or experience.

	Wabi 詫び	**Sabi** 寂び
Current meaning	■ *Rustic simplicity* ■ *Subdued elegance* ■ *Freshness* ■ *Tranquility* ■ *Anomalies or imperfections that are beautiful*	■ *Beauty and calm in what is mature or aged* ■ *Pleasure felt when appreciating the imperfect*
Historical meaning	■ *The solitude of living in nature* ■ *Languishing*	■ *Wizened* ■ *Wilted* ■ *Rusted*

Wabi sabi is a way of seeing life and the universe; its central principle is acceptance of the imperfection and temporary nature of all that resides in the world. It is the beauty of the incomplete, the impermanent and the imperfect.

From a spiritual point of view, it is intricately linked to Zen, as we shall see in the following chapter.

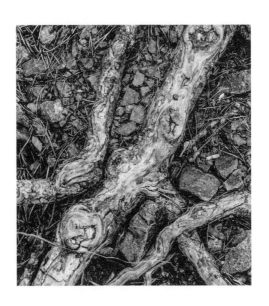

A MEDITATION

it smells of summer,
but by the time I realize this, the trees have turned orange
and fall is here,
suddenly everything is under a white canopy
and winter is here,
the snow melts and the flowers bring color to the world
and spring is here

I live in this hypnotic cycle of the seasons,
but someday I will no longer be here
and they will carry on with their endless transformation,
oblivious to my absence

Zen and Wabi Sabi

"No one enters the same river twice."
—HERACLITUS

There is something inside me that tends to look for a certainty to cling to. Sometimes I even think I cannot be happy or feel safe without it. I secretly wish for the day to come when everything in my life is stable and perfect.

On the other hand, I also know that this paradisiacal state will never come, since the only constant in life is change, the eternal flux of all that exists. There is nothing to cling to, no terra firma to reach, however much our heart longs for it.

For that reason, the only way to be happy is to accept the fact that everything flows relentlessly.

This realization is one of the keys to Buddhist thinking, which in Japan is embodied by Zen, and is regarded as the first key to life.

Buddhism's three keys to life

They are:

1. The impermanence of all living things (in Pāli, *aniccā;* in Japanese, *mujō* 無常).
2. Suffering or impossibility of satisfying all our desires (in Pāli, *dukkha*).
3. Emptiness or nothingness. Absence of the *self*, of the ego.

What does not form part of our self (in Pāli, *śūnyatā*).

Not only are these characteristics shared by all humans, but they are also present in all that exists.

They are three universal truths which are epistemologically self-evident. We need neither science nor anything complicated to demonstrate them. However, some scholars still dispute them, as did others in the past, such as Plato, who made the argument in his innate ideas theory that there is a reality in which nothing changes.

1. Regarding impermanence – the first key to life

In Japanese, we have the expression *shogyō mujō* 諸行無常, which means: *all there is in the world is forever changing, constantly; nothing in the universe is stationary.* Our emotions, thoughts and identity are also always flowing in the time continuum.

We all know what change is. We see it with our eyes and feel it with our emotions, which change from one second to the next. Smells flow, sounds come one after another, the flavors of a delicious dinner continually vary....

Music would cease to be music if it remained stuck in an eternal stationary moment, and the same applies to our lives.

We know that the youthfulness of our bodies is temporary; we will all grow old and die. Impermanence is obviously a part of us and of all that surrounds us.

This mindset isn't limited to Asia. At roughly the same time as the birth of Buddhism, people in other parts of the world started to consider the impermanence of all that surrounds us.

Siddhārtha Gautama was born in the year 480 BC, near the Himalayas, thousands of kilometers from the ancient coastal city of Ephesus, where the pre-Socratic philosopher Heraclitus was born in the year 535 BCE.

One of the fundamental truths of Heraclitus' school of thought is: *panta rei* (Everything flows). Exactly the same as Buddhism's first key to life!

It is what the German philosopher Karl Jaspers called the *Axial Age*, a time of intellectual clarity when humankind in different parts of the world became aware of itself and of its limitations and came to similar conclusions.

This first key to life may be seen in art, which often shows impermanence – the passing of time and the short-lived nature of our existence.

When applied to our day-to-day life, impermanence is an invitation to flow each day and to enjoy the here and now without letting ourselves be weighed down by the past or frightened by the uncertainty of the future.

2. Regarding suffering – the second key to life

In Japanese, we do not have a word to express exactly what the word *dukkha* means. It is not really suffering in the Western sense of the word, of having a really bad time of it because we have been hurt, although it does include that too. Its real meaning is closer to the constant dissatisfaction we feel every day.

Dukkha, dissatisfaction, is the distance that comes between us and that "something more" we are always wishing for. It is as though we are condemned to want something we cannot have, and to never be fully satisfied. This frustration, to a greater or lesser degree, is converted into an emptiness inside us that makes us seek out our next objective.

This may either be something complex, of the existential kind, or something as simple as finishing a meal, feeling satisfied for a brief moment and then right away wanting a piece of chocolate, or wanting to sleep for a while and not being able to do so because there is no futon nearby.

The narrower the gap between our current reality and what we hope to achieve or have, the less *dukkha* or dissatisfaction we will feel, and by extension, the happier we will feel.

To put that into a formula, *happiness is the reality we live in minus what we desire or hope to achieve.*

CURRENT REALITY

|
|
|

(This gap is our dissatisfaction or *dukkha*.
The narrower it is, the less we will suffer)

|
|
|
|

DESIRES
(The perfect reality we imagine.
What we hope to achieve.
What we want but don't have right now)

Happiness equation: *Happiness = Reality – Desires.*

In a best-case scenario, if our desires were equal to zero,

that would mean our happiness would be free of *dukkha* or dissatisfaction.

3. Regarding emptiness – the third key to life

In Japanese, we have the word *ku* 空 to refer to emptiness, both in the literal sense of the word and in the metaphorical sense that is used in Buddhism. But I prefer to use the original word, which in Sanskrit is *śūnyatā*, because its meaning goes further than the Japanese term and is more powerful.

Śūnyatā (Sanskrit) may be translated as "emptiness," "nothing-ness" or "hollow."
It is a term made up of *śūnya*, which means "zero," "nothing," "emptiness," and the affix - *tā*, meaning "that which is."
So, *Śūnyatā* may be translated as "that which is emptiness."

Śūnyatā is a fundamental component of reality and of the cosmos itself, which is largely empty. But it is also an emotional state in which a person no longer feels trapped by worldly desires.

According to some doctrines, *śūnyatā* is everything, since all that exists is empty.

Śūnyatā may also be thought of as a physical and mental state that we humans can reach when we feel things just as they are right now, in the present. That is, our minds are not adding anything at all to reality or eliminating anything whatsoever from it.

Have you ever enjoyed the twilight by the ocean shore? As you observed the sun disappearing, allowing the stars to shine, as you listened to the sound of the surf or breathed in the sea air, did you feel like you were connected to nature? Like you were neither adding nor eliminating anything, simply forming part of it?

If so, it was a *śūnyatā* moment.

The converse is the state we are all continually trapped in, some more so than others, in which we color reality with our emotions and actions.

An everyday example, let's say I have sent a message to a friend and they didn't reply yet. Even though only ten minutes have gone by, I tell myself they probably don't love me anymore. Did they get tired of me? Do they have better friends now? Did they make plans with others? Did I not get invited?

Observe how ego is taking charge of the situation. The questions we ask ourselves are to do with our self-esteem. We are not worried that something might have happened to our friend. What we are really worried about is ourselves, because we feel abandoned.

The ego always tends to come between us and reality, leaving no room for *śūnyatā*.

But after twenty minutes or so our friend replies. It turns out they were reading a book and had left their cell phone charging on the other side of the house....

In the wabi sabi context, as an aesthetic concept applicable to any kind of art, it is essential for a work of art to follow the precepts of *śūnyatā* for it to be considered wabi sabi.

You will be asking yourself: does my work of art have to be empty to be wabi sabi? Not exactly.

Let us say we are creating a sculpture. To have a *śūnyatā* nature, it must fit gracefully into its surroundings, as if it formed part of the whole. The sculpture should not stand apart as though it had its own identity. It will be finished when there is nothing else to add to or take away from it.

The opposite would be a sculpture whose sole purpose is to attract people's attention, or to be spectacular, as though the artist's ego had taken over the work.

Wabi sabi art is the complete opposite. The creator is not to be found in the work—the work is in *śūnyatā* with the universe. It is both art and the universe at one and the same time.

When it comes to our lives, in order to lead a wabi sabi lifestyle, do not add nor eliminate more than is necessary.

For wabi sabi, emptiness, not adding, or nothingness, is just as important as everything else. This is something we can apply equally to creating art and to our lives.

In praise of shadows

We will expand upon this third Buddhist key, especially its implications for art, with a little masterpiece by my compatriot Junichiro Tanizaki. One of Japan's greatest novelists, he is known outside our country for the essay *In Praise of Shadows*, first published in 1933. In this treatise on architectural wabi sabi, Tanizaki reflects on traditional Japanese art and architecture, which were so different from what was practiced in the West.

So, while the West opted for what was bright, polished, straight and harmonious, Japanese architecture played with the minimalism of emptiness—that *śūnyatā* once again— opting for the power of shadow and what was asymmetrical. Japan values an object more if it has a green sheen than if it is gleaming and immaculate.

Let's look at a fragment of that delightful essay:

In reality, the beauty of a Japanese room, produced solely by a play on the degree of opacity of the shadow, needs no other accessory. The Westerner who sees this is surprised by the bareness and believes they are in the presence of nothing more than gray walls bereft of any decoration; this is a perfectly legitimate interpretation from their viewpoint but shows they have completely failed to understand the enigma of the shadow.

Filling oneself with emptiness

Śūnyatā is not only a spiritual or architectural concept, but also a source of inspiration for our life. Put aside days in your calendar with no firm plans and during this time:

- Do whatever you feel like as the day progresses.
- Walk around someplace that has a lot of greenery with someone you love (it may be yourself).
- Close your eyes and concentrate on your breathing for five solid minutes.

Create a *śūnyatā* room in your house:

- Completely empty a room, Put down a carpet and two cushions where you can sit and meditate or read.
- An unwritten rule of this special room is: no electronic device can enter.
- You may buy a thick paintbrush and some ink and sketch a large *ensō* circle on a white parchment (more on the *ensō* in Part II). Hang it in the room next to the two cushions.

The most important lesson that emptiness teaches us is that *you do not need anything to be happy*, other than a little food, water or tea, sleep and the air that you breathe.

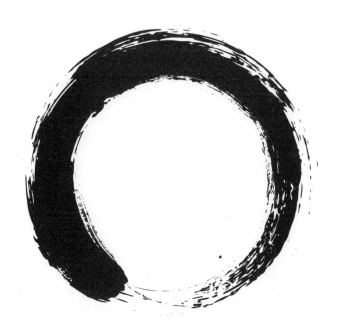

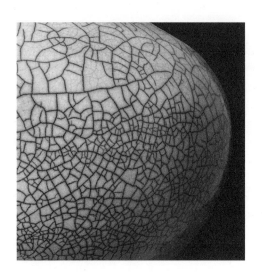

A MEDITATION

My body and mind grow old and change over time.
At the age of ten, I had nothing but curiosity for the world.
At twenty, I wished for action, adventure and passion.
At thirty, for stability and for life to have meaning.
And at forty, I gained wisdom through misadventures.
Having reached fifty,
I now know life is a mystery
and that is precisely what makes it interesting.
More decades will come, or at least I hope so,
since I wish to know what my outlook will be
in each one of them.

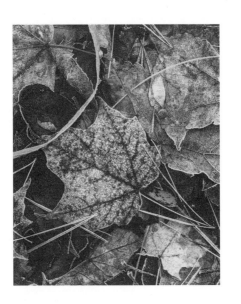

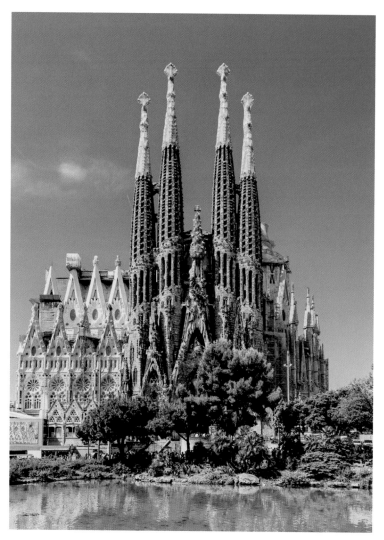

The wabi sabi approach to art and life can be found everywhere in the world. The magnificent basilica Sagrada Família in Barcelona is a mix of Gothic and Modern forms, bringing together old and new, belonging fully to neither one nor the other. This passionate endeavor by Catalan architect Antoni Gaudí, whose work on the project began in 1883, was only partially finished at the time of his death in 1926, and remains a work in progress.

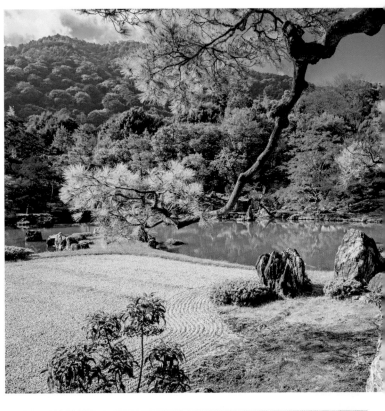

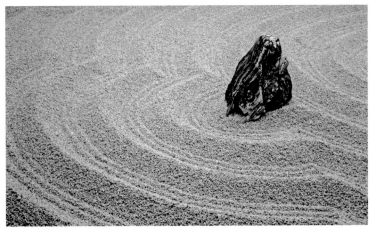

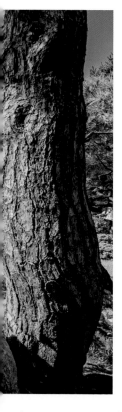

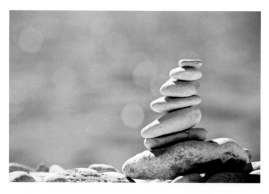

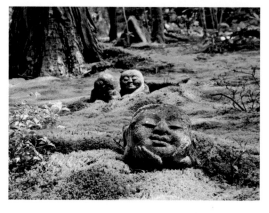

[CLOCKWISE FROM TOP LEFT] At the Tenryu-ji Temple in Arashiyama, Japan, we see greens, golds and reds as summer gradually cedes to fall. Transitional times have a beauty all their own, as we prepare to say a grateful farewell to what has passed and look forward to what is to come.

Stacked stones are a common symbol associated with Zen. The placing of the stones is an act of prayer or meditation, and each stone can be imbued with meaning. The structure is held together only by the balancing of the stones. Eventually, nature will dismantle the altar. Everything happens as it is meant to.

Almost as if they're "resting in nature," tranquil faces at the Sanzen-in Temple (Ohara, Kyoto) are a reminder of our ultimate relationship with the earth. These childlike faces represent Warabe-Jizō, protector of children and travelers.

In temple gardens, raking the gravel of a rock garden is a daily practice, as in this garden at Daitokuji Temple in Kyoto. Circular patterns, linear patterns, and patterns like the one you see here all represent both the constancy and the inconstancy of nature. The stones remain steadfast, even though they too change with time, while the "water" flows around them.

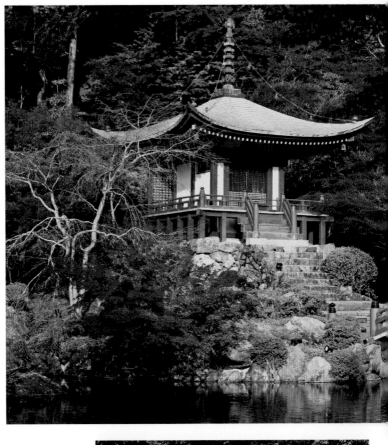

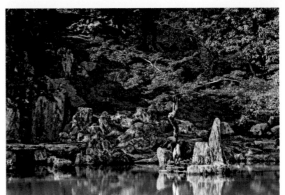

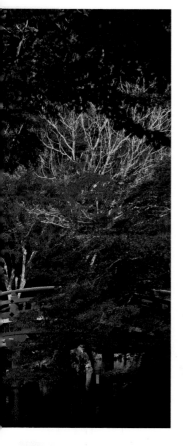

The spirit of wabi sabi is in full harmony with the cycle of the seasons. Here, fall comes to the garden of the Daigoji Temple in Kyoto. The beauty of the leaves as they reach the end of their cycle is unique from one year to the next. It tugs at the soul while it captivates the eye, even as we look forward to the blossoming of sakura in the following spring.

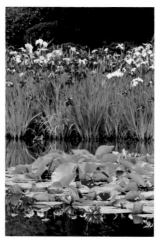

Rock, tree, water, summer and fall, darkness and light—as seen here, you sometimes can have everything at once, for a short time. Such moments will pass, just as the leaves on the trees will eventually fall into the water below, so be open and present to these moments when they come.

Each season has stages within it, and all of them have beauty— even that moment just after the last leaves have fallen and snow has yet to come. At the Heian Jingū Shrine in Kyoto, early summer is the time for irises and water lilies. Japanese irises thrive during the rainy season, and they stand out against gray and sunny skies alike. Water lilies, rising from murky depths, are proof that there's great beauty to be found in mud.

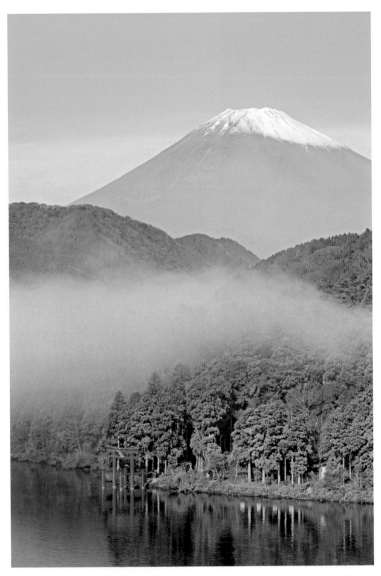

The most iconic symbol of Japan, Mt. Fuji is an active volcano that can destroy utterly, yet it is teeming with life. Connecting earth to heaven, it is a place held scared, yet its environment is disrupted by human activity year after year. It is steadfast, but not unchanging. And by many people from the birthplace of wabi sabi, the mountain is revered as the very soul of Japan.

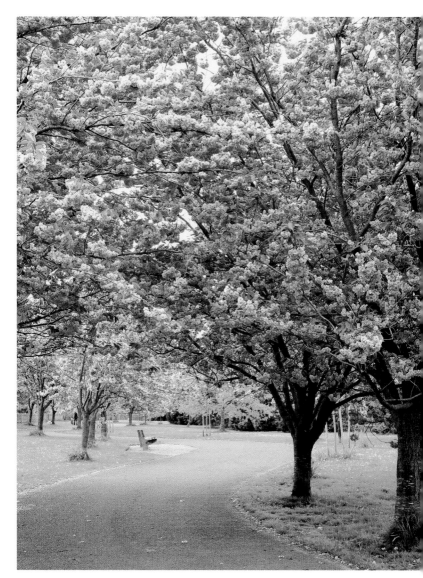

The flowering time of the sakura is glorious but brief, precious because it is ephemeral. As a symbol of friendship between nations, this tree is celebrated in festivals the world over. In Japan, the entire season is a festival.

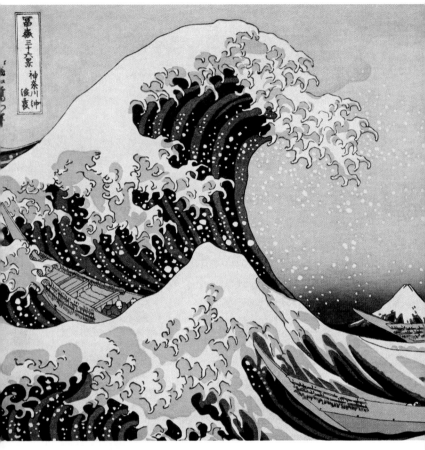

For centuries Mt. Fuji has inspired artists from many parts of the world. Hokusai's "The Great Wave Off Kanagawa" is one of the world's most beloved works of art, replicated in ways too numerous to count. Yet many viewers are unaware that its origins lie in a series called *Thirty-six Views of Mt. Fuji*. And sure enough, the mountain stands in the background, overlooking this scene of potential destruction. The sea and the mountain—nature showing its presence and its power in two different forms.

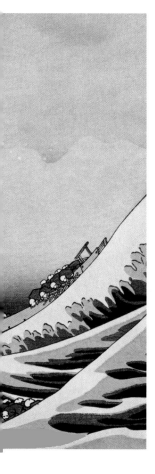

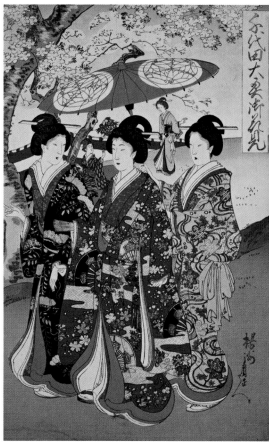

Hanami is the cherry blossom season's tradition of taking time to go out and commune with the trees, and share meals beneath their branches with family and friends. It is an example of how deeply the spirit of wabi sabi is ingrained in Japanese culture. Experience the beauty of each season while it lasts—the season is here and gone, and when it returns, its beauty will be different from what it was the year before. Above, a detail from *Chiyoda Ooku Ohanami* by Toyohara Chikanobu (1838-1912) gives a taste of the sort of salute and celebration that continues to this day.

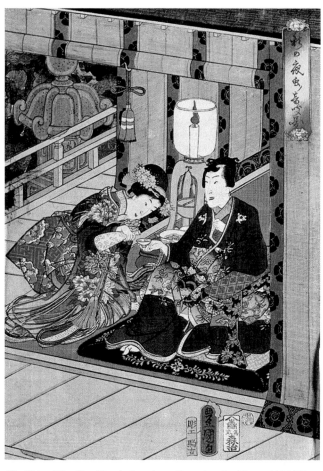

The Tale of Genji, written in the eleventh century by Murasaki Shikibu, is acknowledged as the world's first novel. It documents the title character's many rises and falls, triumphs and failures, qualities and shortcomings—what he has learned and what he has failed to learn— over the course of more than a thousand pages. As we know from our enjoyment of novels past and present, it is the character's mixture of light and shade that gives the novel its resonance. It is his flaws, quirks, pleasures and failures that secure our sympathy. Our understanding and enjoyment of the imperfect extends not only to the natural world, but to the human one as well. And although he is undeniably a flawed character, Genji has a gift for living in the moment. In this detail from an 1860 print by Kunisada, Genji enjoys the sight of fall foliage while a young maid serves him sake.

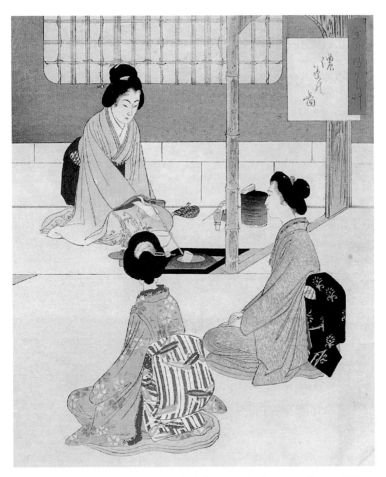

As the tea ceremony became increasingly important in Japanese life, so did the frequency of its depictions in Japanese art increase. The print above is one of myriad prints of the ceremony performed for one person or many, and by the highest and lowest people in society.

In this print from the series *A Tea Ceremony Periwinkle* by Toshikata Mizuno (1866-1908), the hostess prepares tea in the sight of her guests. The concept of wabi sabi has its origins in the tea ceremony. Wabi sabi is present not only in the simplicity and neatness of the setting, and the imperfections in the tea bowls. It is in the act of making, giving and receiving tea with a full and pure heart. It is in the feeling of serenity with one's self and the other participants. In a ceremony well performed and attended, the participants feel the *wabi*—the serene melancholy in the beauty and transience of the present moment.

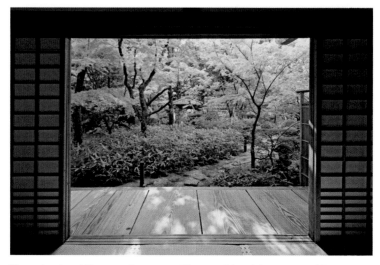

The natural world is never far removed from traditional Japanese architecture. The Kotoin Temple in Kyoto opens wide to the garden outside.

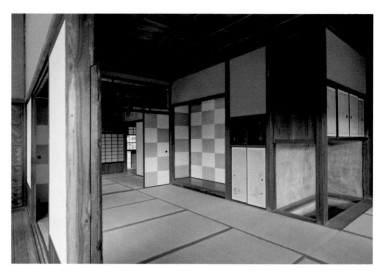

The Katsura Imperial Villa is both rustic and artful, with its checkered *fusuma* (sliding doors) that allow rooms to expand and air to circulate, and give easy access to the garden outside.

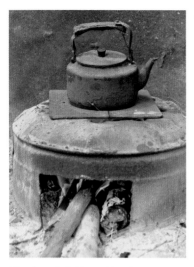

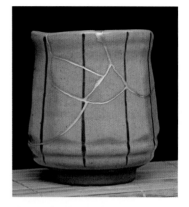

Weathered, flaking, with a few dents here and there, its handle repaired, this kettle has seen long service, and it continues to serve. When it is worn or broken beyond repair, it may rest on a shelf in the home, an old friend appreciated for what it gave. In wabi sabi, that which is worth having appreciates rather than depreciates over time, not because it is well-preserved, but because age, wear and long use have increased its beauty and meaning.

Kintsugi (gold joinery) is a slow and mindful process, involving many steps and a lot of waiting before moving from one step to the next. The gold highlights and celebrates the break that leads to the repair, as well as the repair itself. The repair, performed with love and care, creates something new out of what which was broken, something even more precious than the original.

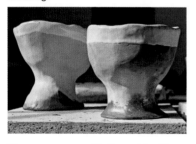

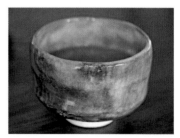

These cups exemplify the wabi sabi aspect of *raku* pottery. Hand-shaped rather than thrown, traditionally fired at lower temperatures, then cooled outside the kiln once the glazes have melted, a *raku* piece's final form is wonderfully unpredictable. [Right] Prized and loved for their irregularities, *raku* tea bowls remain a part of the Japanese tea ceremony to this day.

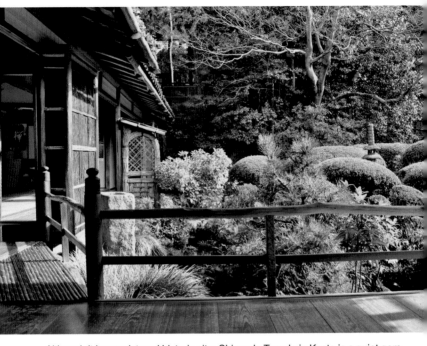

Although it is a registered historic site, Shisendo Temple in Kyoto is a quiet gem. Rustic from its gates to its gardens, it is an excellent example of wabi sabi architecture, deferring to nature and softening the lines between indoors and out.

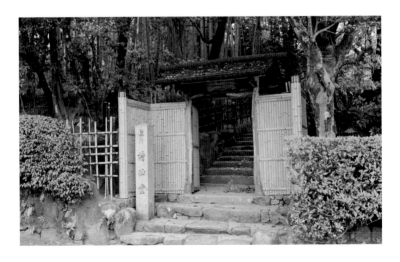

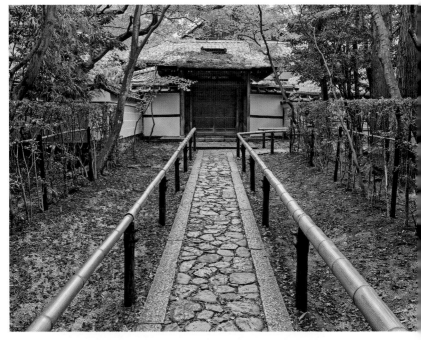

The Daitokuji Temple in Kyoto is like a complex of gardens with buildings attached. The buildings are designed to make the gardens accessible from within. Pathways throughout the complex offer a sort of "moving contemplation."

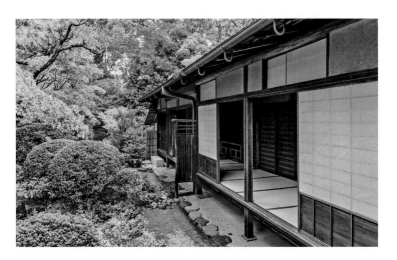

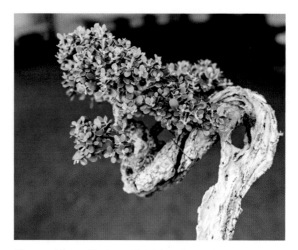

The art of *bonsai* is the artificial dwarfing and arrangement of a tree's form, resulting in trunks and roots that are twisted or gnarled, and branches that may be sparse or barren. While this is in many ways the antithesis of letting nature take its course, it venerates the laws of nature by replicating old age, imperfection and the impact of the elements.

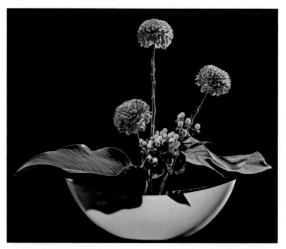

Ikebana is the Japanese art of using the line, form, color and the intrinsic qualities of flowers and foliage to express meaning. It uses no more or less than is needed to complete the thought. Balance is found not through symmetry or bulk, but through the flowers, twigs and leaves themselves.

Don't Be Too Hard on Yourself and on Others

"None of us live in an objective world,
but instead in a subjective world
that we ourselves have given meaning to.
The world you see is different from the one I see,
and it's impossible to share your world with anyone else."
—ICHIRO KISHIMI

Japanese culture is well known for its work ethic, summed up by the expression *ganbarimasu* 頑張ります, which translates as "doing it the best you can." If we analyze the term, 頑 means "stubbornness" and could mean "stretch," so the expression may literally be understood to mean "stretch your stubbornness as far as possible."

This key principle of life is especially useful for students and athletes, whom we encourage before an exam or competition with a "Ganbatte kudasai," which means something along the lines of "strive to do it the best you can."

While it's a good concept for maintaining focus and effort, "ganbarimasu" can turn against us if we distort it or live too strictly by it in our daily lives, since life is not a race and it is impossible for us to even aspire to perfection, as wabi sabi philosophy reminds us.

Antithesis of wabi sabi philosophy Aspiring to perfection	Wabi sabi philosophy Accepting imperfection
Adulation of what is invincible	Respect for what is fragile
Feeling of stress because we allow our feelings to control us	Dynamic calmness, observing what we feel
Perfection	Imperfection
Magnanimousness	Modesty
Adding more than is necessary and finally ending up being false	Honesty
Trying or hoping for things to go on forever	Accepting that every-thing is impermanent
Thinking logically about the past and the future as though they were something fixed and im-movable	Being focused on the here and now
Haste	Pauses
Mental confusion	Mental clarity

Same firmament, different stars

It is good to try hard when we are trying to reach the summit of a mountain, even spurring on our fellow climbers, but to keep this spirit up in situations where it makes no sense only achieves the opposite effect; fatigue and demotivation in others and disappointment and resentment within oneself.

This is relevant in the sphere of friendships and even more so when it comes to couples.

Apart from being useless, hoping that our friends will meet our expectations is a sure-fire path to loneliness, since we will get upset with them one by one and end up losing them. Expressions like, "*If I were you, I'd have done this or the other,*" when we feel let down because we were hoping for a different response from them, in reality encapsulate a profound ignorance of the individuality of the human condition.

No two people think or react alike, because each person is at a different point on their journey. It is impossible to be in anyone else's shoes because each person has their own place from where they observe the universe.

To make use of that simile, it is as though each person lives on a planet in a different galaxy. All of us are surrounded by the same firmament of stars but the configurations change depending on where the observer happens to be.

The galaxy we inhabit is made up of our innate character, the family into which we were born and our experiences throughout life. This combination of things conditions our outlook and places each of us in a corner of the world where we alone dwell.

How are others supposed to react according to our wishes, which are often not even verbalized, if they live in a different galaxy with another sky chart?

This is just what happens—with more serious consequences- when one half of a couple wishes to mold the other for their benefit. Frictions multiply and may lead to a breakup. Each person's character is molded in its own way and is a unique piece with its own cracks and irregularities. If they were to disappear, the person would cease to be themselves.

The wabi sabi of love implies loving those characteristics that make that person unique and only altering – by mutual consent—what jeopardizes the bond.

Does the truth even exist?

In 1950, in one of his most famous movies, *Rashōmon*, Akira Kurosawa told a remarkable tale, set in twelfth-century Kyoto.

The authorities have to solve the murder of a man that took place in a forest close to a ruined temple. The investigators come across four completely different versions of the events: those of the dead man's wife, the bandit, the only witness and even the murdered man himself, who describes what happened through a medium.

After hearing the four wildly differing accounts, they reach the conclusion that it is impossible to know the truth.

In the 1960s, the hippiedom and psychedelia that drank from the mysticism of India went still further, going so far as to doubt the very existence of reality itself. As the Beatles sang in "Strawberry Fields Forever," nothing is real.

And here in the twenty-first century, in *3-Iron*, a movie by Kim Ki Duk about an otherworldly motorcyclist who moves from one house to another, living in them while their owners are away, the following phrase appears at the end:

"It's hard to tell whether the world we live in is a reality or a dream."

Be the best imperfect person you can be

If each person has their own truth and we cannot even be certain of the reality we believe ourselves to be living in, what sense is there in having certainties about how things are or how they should be?

Maybe it would be more sensible to rediscover the wisdom of the old Greek masters and recognize that the wisest person is the one who knows they know nothing, since in that principle of ignorance lies the seed of all future growth.

By approaching life from the wabi sabi perspective, we embrace the utter uncertainty of existence, along with the mystery of our own abilities.

When a little girl sits at the piano for the first time and her fingers coax sounds out of the keys, it is impossible to know whether the game will come to little else or if, with the passing of time, her passion for playing will rapidly burgeon until it makes her into a virtuoso performer, in demand in the world's best concert halls.

That is the magic of humankind, which is imperfect but at the same time has the potential for *everything*.

On that subject, Doctor Shoma Morita, a contemporary of Freud and the creator of a life goal-based therapy, influenced by Zen Buddhism, stated the following:

Give up on yourself. Begin taking action now, while being neurotic or imperfect, or a procrastinator, or unhealthy, or lazy, or any other label by which you inaccurately describe yourself. Go ahead and be the best imperfect person you can be and get started on those things you want to accomplish before you die.

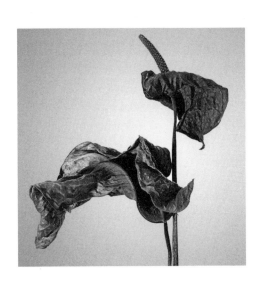

A MEDITATION

the branches of the keyaki in my garden
sway in the dawn breeze
I want to be like that tree:
to have deep roots
but to bend my branches
when my life is battered
by the storm

keyaki: large deciduous tree native to Japan

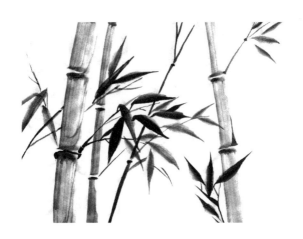

Lessons from Nature

"What a strange thing!
To be alive
beneath cherry blossoms."
—KOBAYASHI ISSA

As we saw in the first chapters of this book, nature is the great master of wabi sabi philosophy, because it is the inspiration for the beauty of that which is imperfect, incomplete and perishable.

Nothing is completely geometrical or symmetrical—that is a human obsession—but nature finds its own beauty in that which is irregular.

Nothing is finished, nor will it ever be, since the idea of "a finished work" is a human obsession. Nature is an endless work in progress, like the life of a human being while they journey through this life.

Nothing is everlasting—the cycle of births and deaths is all that is eternal. Life endlessly renews itself and us with it, inside and out.

Nature is a great master but we humans have distanced ourselves from her so much that we have forgotten her humble lessons. We shall rediscover them through the diaries of different hermits.

Lazy philosophy notes

Among the Japanese texts that best reflect the spirit of wabi sabi are the so-called *Essays in Idleness* that the monk Yoshida Kenkō wrote between 1330 and 1332. He wrote them on pieces of paper he would stick to the walls of his secluded cabin.

It is said that years later a friend of his devoted himself to carefully peeling off those bits of paper and, by gathering 243 fragments, rescued one of the most brilliant works of Japanese literature.

Tsurezuregusa, as these essays are known in Japanese, speak of the fleeting nature of all things. Kenkō's writings also put across the simplicity, humility and naturalness that are characteristic of Zen. They urge the reader to take advantage of every waking breath through contemplation of nature and of their own mind.

Let us take a look at some fragments from this compendium of inspiration that transmit the essence of wabi sabi:

"In all things, uniformity is undesirable. Leaving something incomplete... gives one the feeling that through this imperfection the life of living things is extended."

In contrast with the modern obsession with order – perhaps to compensate for inner disorder and disquiet – this fourteenth century monk praised the value of that which is incomplete:

Leaving something incomplete makes life interesting. It is said that even when building the imperial palace, some corner is always left unfinished. And in the writings of the old spiritual masters, there are always chapters and parts missing.

Non-completion and disorder is also present in our everyday life, where we never know what might happen, but Yoshida Kenkō sees this as a value: *"Life's most precious gift is uncertainty."*

This component of poverty and parsimony, which is ever present in wabi sabi, is a hallmark of *Essays in Idleness,* where the poet points out that none of the sages of antiquity had possessions, and he gives the extreme example of the Chinese hermit Xu You:

He had not a single possession in the world. He would even scoop up water with his hands, until a friend gave him a hollowed-out pumpkin. But one day after hanging it from a branch, he heard the wind make it rattle. As the noise bothered him, he cast the pumpkin away and carried on drinking by cupping his hands. How pure and free was that man's heart!

Yoshida Kenkō talks of another man who was so free that, when being held prisoner, he stated that the only thing he would regret leaving when he died was the sky.

Hymn to life from a hut
Essays in Idleness is a classic of the *zuihitsu* genre, a spontaneous way of writing made popular in the eleventh century by Sei Shonagon, the author of *The Pillow Book*, which recounts her everyday experiences at the empress's court.

Another well-known diary is *Hōjōki,* sometimes translated as *Hymn to Life from a Hut.* Written in 1212 by the hermit poet Kamo no Chōmei, it explains his life in a ten-foot square shack, from where he observed nature and life.

The beginning of this short essay is renowned in Japanese literature. This is how it talks of the passing of time and the temporariness of life:

The current of the flowing river does not cease, and yet the water is not the same water as before. The foam that floats on stagnant pools is illusionary; now vanishing, now forming, it never stays the same for long.

The account shows Kamo no Chōmei knew how to live in the purest wabi sabi spirit:

Now I dwell in my quiet home. It is merely a ten-foot square cabin, but I love it. When I go to the capital for something, I may feel ashamed of my beggar's appearance, but upon returning I feel pity for the people I see there, so absorbed by a life of worry about wealth and honor, so busy. If you doubt what I say, think about the fish and the birds: the fish are always in the water and yet they do not grow tired of it. Although if you are not a fish, you probably won't understand that; as for the birds, they pine for the forest. Although if you are not a bird, you probably won't understand their reasons either. My feelings toward my quiet home imply the same thing. Who can understand it if they have never tried it?

My life, just like the waning moon, is about to end. The remaining days are few in number.

Life in the woods
The Western equivalent of these essays on austere life, the result of life in a cabin, came in the modern era, with the ex-

60

perience of Henry David Thoreau. After an intense social life in Concord, where he had his neighbor Ralph Waldo Emerson as a mentor, he decided to build a hut with his own hands near Walden Pond.

This American philosopher, the father of civil disobedience, abandoned the hustle and bustle of city life so as not to be like "the mass of men who live lives of quiet desperation."

He considered that urban idleness had cut him off from the heart of life, preventing him from writing authentically. In his own words: "*How vain it is to sit down to write when you have not stood up to live.*"

He would remain there for two years, two months and two days, while he put down in writing what would end up being the most famous essay of his time, published in 1854 as *Walden* or *Life in the Woods*.

As an example of the many lessons the American author drew from nature, we find these transcendental reflections on the song of the thrush in his *Notes on Birds of New England*:

> *…In the thrush's [note], though heard at noon, there is the liquid coolness of things that are just drawn from the bottom of springs. The thrush alone declares the immortal wealth and vigor that is in the forest. Here is a bird in whose strain the story is told, though Nature waited for the science of aesthetics to discover it to man. Whenever a man hears it, he is young, and Nature is in her spring. Wherever he hears it, it is a new world and a free country, and the gates of heaven are not shut against him. Most other birds sing from the level of my ordinary cheerful hours—a carol; but this bird never*

> *fails to speak to me out of an ether purer than that I breathe, of immortal beauty and vigor. He deepens the significance of all things seen in the light of his strain. He sings to make men take higher and truer views of things. He sings to amend their institutions; to relieve the slave on the plantation and the prisoner in his dungeon, the slave in the house of luxury and the prisoner of his own low thoughts.*

Thoreau, however, was not a typical hermit. We know that inside his tiny cabin there were three chairs and when asked about them, he replied: "One is for solitude, two for friendship, three for society."

Although he would end up returning to Concord after finishing his long retreat, what he learned from nature enlightened the rest of his life, giving his heart peace.

When he became seriously ill at the age of forty-four and entered his final days, his aunt, who looked after him, asked him if he had made peace with God, to which he replied: "I didn't know we had fallen out."

On 6th May 1862 he uttered one last phrase on his deathbed: "Now comes good sailing."

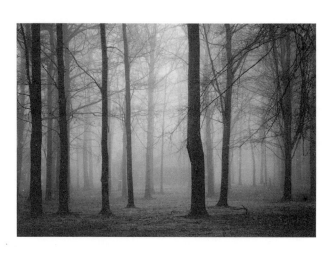

II
Wabi Sabi in Art

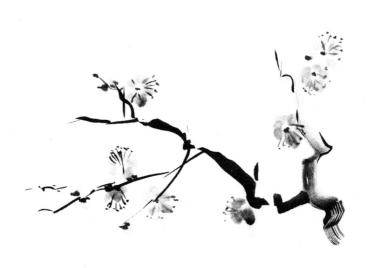

A MEDITATION

The crows perch on the maple tree branches,
their cawing echoing around the hillside.
When the evening sun
is reflected in the pond, I wonder:
What is more beautiful?
The echo or the original sound?
The sun or the reflected sunbeams?

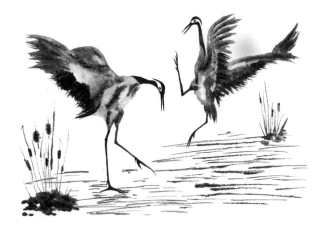

Principles of Wabi Sabi in the Japanese Arts

"As imperfect humans
we are allergic to what is perfect.
If something is perfect from start to finish
there is no suggestion of the infinite."
—YANAGI SŌETSU

My freelance lifestyle gives me the time to travel freely. Whenever I can, I like to set out without a specific destination, in search of little-known corners of our islands.

A short time ago, I accepted an offer to visit the Daijoji Zen Temple. Twenty monks live there, who begin their day with a two-hour meditation session at 4.30 a.m.

I awoke one hour before dawn in a *ryokan*[1] near the temple. After crossing the shadowy woods, I reached the black gate that marks the entrance to the complex. Legend has it the black *mon*[2] was the first thing they built before deciding to establish the temple.

The wood of the mon is so dark it looks as though it is going to swallow up the forest, like some kind of black hole. Moss grows on top of the gate and even plants, whose offshoots and leaves make the mon appear to be wearing a straw hat.

---

[1] A traditional Japanese hotel
[2] Entrance gate in a Buddhist temple

A little further along, after crossing the entrance, there is an enormous bell and perpendicular to it is a log, which is used to strike it. I halted there for a few moments to observe the *dharma* wheel, inscribed both on the rusty metal of the bell and on the log. The *dharma* wheel always makes me reflect on my mortality as a human being.

When I die, both the bell and the black *mon* will still be there, living in harmony with the forest wilderness.

Once there, I meditated with the Daijoji monks. As I was not used to meditating for so long at a time, my legs and back hurt by the end of the two hours.

When the meditation finished, one of the monks struck the bell, and the sound of it reverberating inside me made my senses become as one with the universe for a brief instant. A strange space had been created between moments, as though the bell had suspended the passing of time.

"Is this happiness?" I wondered.

Then they invited me to eat *shōjin ryōri*[3] and drink tea with them.

---

[3] A specific type of vegan Buddhist cuisine

Dharmachackra or dharma wheel

Only in the equilibrium of all the elements of the *dharma* wheel may enlightenment be attained. Each one of the wheel's eight vertices represents one of the eight divisions of the Noble Eightfold Path:

1. Death is not the end, and our actions in this life have consequences after we die.
2. It is important to intend to contemplate impermanence and the inevitability of suffering.
3. You should not lie.
4. You should not kill nor inflict harm on others.
5. We should only possess what is essential for living and nothing else.
6. We need to awaken our consciousness, without letting ourselves be seized by sensorial desires, envy or jealousy.
7. We should use meditation.
8. Finally, we come to *Samadhi*: the state a person attains when they feel their body and mind are becoming at one with the universe.

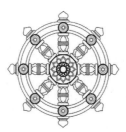

The *dharma* wheel is a symbol that joins cultures and religions. It is shared by Buddhism, Hinduism, and Jainism. [image by FreeeSVG.org]

The *raku* soul

Days later, I went to Nagano to visit the Sunritz Hattori art museum, which is on the shore of Lake Suwa. They keep a *chawan*[4] there which is listed as a national treasure. It is a *raku* piece called "Mount Fuji" created by Honami Kōetsu in the early seventeenth century.

Raku is a Japanese pottery technique that arose in the sixteenth century and which uses relatively low oven temperatures.

Honami Kōetsu's white *raku* piece is considered an historic work of art because it contains the very essence of wabi sabi. On seeing this little bowl, which is not even four inches high, I sensed my heart swelling as it felt the power and humility of the piece.

My vision blurred and my emotions overflowed upon observing Honami Kōetsu's "Mount Fuji."

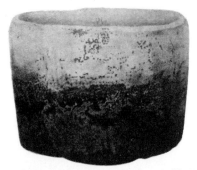

Ceramic *raku* bowl called "Mount Fuji" created by Honami Kōetsu. It is listed as a national treasure by the Japanese government. [Photo from the National Diet Library]

---

[4] Tea bowl

Wabi sabi rebels against the modernity that seeks in vain to create perfectly flat surfaces and symmetrical shapes, elements which aid mass production. Unlike the latter, *raku* objects are unique – no one can copy or even imitate Honami Kōetsu's "Mount Fuji."

Going from the mountain contained within the gentle irregularity of a little bowl to one you can actually walk on, that very day I climbed Kirigamine, whose literal translation is "among the mists." The hiking route to it begins right next to the museum. It was a fine day and from the summit I was able to look upon the Japanese Alps mountain range. Then I sat down on a rock to eat an *onigiri* (rice ball) and drink a little green tea.

Sitting at the summit of Kirigamine, I was overwhelmed by a feeling of joy and connection to nature, while reminiscences of Honami Kōetsu's white *raku* endured within me. To my heart, the bowl and Nagano's natural surroundings were not separate entities but integral parts of a single experience.

The essence of nature and wabi sabi art is the same.

The wabi sabi architect

Two years ago, I went on a long trip around Europe. I walked until exhausted around the historical city centers, admiring the facades which are designed down to the last detail.

Despite this, straight lines dominate, and curves only appear when necessary. The European architect seeks perfection, creating pristine spaces, which are almost worthy of the gods.

I noticed a hint of wabi sabi in the churches and cathedrals, as though they wanted to escape from the restrictions and could allow themselves a certain mystical degree of madness.

But it was not until I arrived in Barcelona that I came across the artist who truly connects the West and the East: Antoni Gaudí.

The Sagrada Familia, the Casa Milà and the Park Güell are one hundred percent wabi sabi.

The first, with its impossible curves and telluric presence, seems to have emerged from the entrails of the Earth, like a volcano or a mountain. It aims to be a work of art created by nature itself rather than by humans.

Gaudí was not trying to outdo nature but to create art embodying the essence of the natural world. He did not want to impose his ego on the world by having something superior to what Creation had built.

In common with the Catalan architect, Japanese Shintoist sanctuaries and Buddhist temples do not try to impose something artificial either, rather they integrate with the surrounding nature. I compare these sacred Shintoist spaces with the Park Güell, where nature and artificiality merge into one element.

We will now go back to the bowl that served to illustrate wabi sabi in art, to see some of its characteristics.

Organic texture: *yūki tekusucha* 有機テクスチャ

The bowls made with the *raku* technique are characterized by their organic texture. Depending on the scale at which you observe the object, its appearance changes dynamically.

Perfectly flat surfaces, with a uniform color, are always similar, regardless of whether you are looking at them from ten inches or ten feet away. Flat and perfect things only exist in the artificial world.

Only works of art with irregular organic textures may be considered wabi sabi. There is nothing that attracts the human eye more than flaws, and nothing that is duller than monotony.

And not only sight but the rest of human senses are more sensitive when there is some kind of change. We lose our sense of smell when we get used to an odor. If we hear a tune which keeps repeating the same four notes, it will become tiresome and repetitive. As for touch, if someone who has never caressed us before touches us, it will feel quite different from what we feel with the caress of someone who has been with us for years.

We can feel whatever changes or is dynamic more intensely. Organic textures are the true expression of continuous change.

Simplicity: *kanso* 簡素

This aesthetic and spiritual virtue aims to achieve optimal results using as little as possible. Eliminate all that which is unimportant or superfluous to leave space for what is essential.

Do not add anything that is not strictly necessary.

We can only attain *kanso* by excluding everything that is not essential, like a beautiful sculpture that has thrown off the rock that enclosed it, like a stone cocoon.

Simplicity is the ultimate sophistication. Oscar Wilde said that "simple pleasures are the last refuge of the complex," and there is certainly a clear link between simplicity and sophistication.

Young poets, for instance, often write lengthy verses to express quite simple ideas. Due to their inexperience, they get bogged down in unnecessary complexity.

The elderly poetry master, on the other hand, is capable of

expressing something extraordinarily complex, such as the meaning of life, with three simple *haiku* phrases.

Asymmetry and flaws: *fukinsei* 不均整

The meaning of *fukinsei* encompasses both asymmetry and irregularity in general. An oft-used example of this characteristic of wabi sabi art is the *ensō* circle.

This circle, which is practiced by calligraphy masters, is never symmetrical. On the contrary, the spontaneity of the brushstroke must be visible. Nor is the circle closed, since the *ensō* symbolizes the incompleteness of all that exists, the pure spirit of wabi sabi.

Well-executed, naturally flowing asymmetry, is beautiful, since only through calmness is the artist able to find the balance within chaos – that is the essence of *fukinsei*.

Naturalness: *shizen* 自然

For a Japanese, everything is more beautiful when it bears the marks of the passing of time. In fact, wounds or flaws distinguish what is unique from what is commonplace. This is equally applicable to the wrinkles or scars of a person and to the rust on a saucepan or kettle.

What is natural and unpretentious is wabi sabi.

An old man or woman with deep wrinkles and a still-adolescent smile is the pinnacle of wabi sabi beauty.

Western art *Seeking perfection*	Wabi sabi art *Accepting imperfection*
Symmetry	Asymmetry
Search for perfection	Imperfections are embraced
Proportions following Greco-Roman ideals	Proportions are unimportant
Refinement	Roughness
Complexity	Simplicity
There is an attempt to impress the onlooker more than is strictly necessary	Only those elements that are necessary are kept
Artificiality	Appreciation of what is natural
Imposing and spectacular	Intimate
Intellectual and rational	Intuitive
Magnificent	Austere
Sublime	Modest
Static	Dynamic
Limits itself to representing something finite	Evokes the infinite
Regular	Irregular and random
Brilliant and pristine	Used, rusty

Your first wabi sabi work of art

According to the *mingei* philosophy of my compatriot Yanagi Muneyoshi, what any person creates, without any need for them to be an artist, is in principle beyond beauty and ugliness.

I challenge you to create a wabi sabi object following the *mingei* philosophy. Yanagi Muneyoshi's rules are:

- It must be handmade.
- It must be made with inexpensive materials.
- Anybody should be able to appreciate or use it.
- It must be representative in some way of the region where it was created.

Following Yanagi's inspiration, this is what I did:

1. I bought a wooden board in a secondhand store.
2. I polished it to restore it but not to remove its imperfections. On the contrary, I worked to make them stand out more, leaving the texture exposed. In this way, I managed to get one of the knots to be the wood's main feature.
3. I put the board in a corner of my tatami room and placed a small vase on top of it containing a bunch of flowers I had picked on a hill near my house.

My little *mingei* work therefore followed the principles of wabi sabi: simplicity (*kanso*), naturalness (*shizen*), asymmetry (*fukinsei*) and organic texture (*yūki tekusucha*).

A MEDITATION

I walk along the roji to the teahouse.
The path narrows as I draw closer
to the door where the ceremony awaits me.
As I go on, something changes inside of me.
I remain in this world but at the same time
I feel I am traveling to a place
that is faraway but very close to my heart.
When I finally arrive and take off my shoes,
I am no longer the same person
who began to walk along the roji.

roji: a narrow garden path with stepping stones that indicates the way to a traditional Japanese teahouse

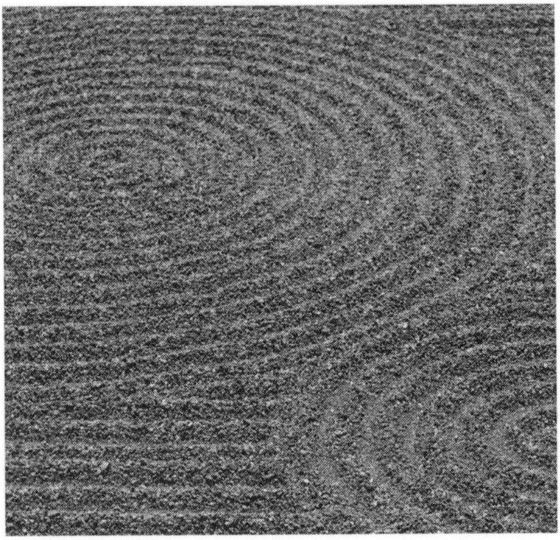

The Beauty of Melancholy

*"Put your soul in the palm of my hand
for me to look at,
like a crystal jewel."
I'll sketch it in words..."*
—YASUNARI KAWABATA

Wabi sabi is present in the melancholic feeling where the beauty and the fleeting nature of life converge. We sense it in an autumnal photograph, when contemplating the trees whose branches have become almost bare. We also sense it when we experience something wonderful that inundates our soul and that we would like to hold onto forever, which is impossible.

It has happened to everyone at one time or another.

I recall how on one occasion I traveled to the island of Koh Tao, in the south of Thailand. After a week relaxing in a bungalow by the emerald sea, I took the evening boat to the mainland, from where my return train to Bangkok would depart.

I was standing on the ferry deck, when we passed through an inlet full of fishing boats just before reaching port. The sight of those traditional vessels, beacons blazing in the sunset, captivated me. There were families having dinner on deck, youths carrying sacks of provisions or newly repaired nets and children with their feet hanging over the water.

Faced with this bucolic picture postcard scene, I was overwhelmed by a feeling of happiness mixed with a trace of sadness. In the deepest part of my being, I knew I would never return to that place, whose name I can no longer even remember. That is to say, at the same time as I was gaining that experience, I was about to lose it, and that is what caused my melancholy.

This is a typically wabi sabi feeling.

A receding sea wake

Kamo no Chōmei, the Japanese poet and hermit, who died in 1216, explained the meaning of *wabi* way back in his time, and did so in the following terms:

"Wabi is the feeling the sky gives us on a fall afternoon, the melancholy of color, when all sounds have been silenced. Those moments in which for some reason the mind cannot explain, tears begin to fall uncontrollably."

Perhaps what the mind cannot explain is the certainty of the impermanence of life, like the scene I have just narrated, which in turn includes our own impermanence. Knowing we are birds of passage brings us this melancholic perception of beauty and of life.

In moments like this, we feel that the happiness that comes to us through perception and our personal experiences is a loan, something that sooner rather than later will be snatched away from us. We realize that it will never be entirely ours and that is what increases its worth.

And what of *wabi*'s fellow traveler in this concept?

The word *sabi* is used to describe the austere beauty of ancient Japanese poetry, of the haiku that with just three brushstrokes captures the sparrow looking for food among the fallen autumnal leaves.

Going even further back in time, as far back as the eighth century there lived a Buddhist monk called Mansei who practiced an innovative kind of poetry in the spirit of wabi sabi.

One of the few remaining fragments of his work goes:
To what should I compare this world?
To a white wake left by a boat receding in the dawn?

What use is melancholy?

In a society where it appears we are forced to be constantly happy, and where melancholy is suffocated through medication, wabi sabi provides us with a profound outlook on the reality surrounding us. This reality is neither uniquely joyful nor sad, but includes both emotions at once, as we have just seen. That is where its beauty lies.

Every loss carries an inherent gain: the valuing of what we have left even more than we did before. When someone gets over a difficult illness, perhaps their strength has lessened, but they acquire a greater appreciation of life. Especially if they have been at death's door, they now know the value of each and every moment and are eager to enjoy every single one.

The same happens to us when leaving a funeral. As we are reminded of the transitory nature of life, we determine to live it in a nobler way, so as not to exit this world leaving our bill with happiness outstanding.

That is one of the benefits of melancholy. As we become aware of the transient nature of things, we confer greater importance on them. At the same time, it brings us a more profound outlook on reality, which also happens with art.

We may say that a piece of music full of subtle melancholy is more profound than an upbeat military march, in the same way that it would be hard to write a good novel about a couple whose love for one another is unhindered or about a perfectly happy family.

In fact, a study published in the journal *Perspectives on Psychological Science* (vol. 2, no. 4, December 1, 2007) showed that people who are overly satisfied with their life lack self-criticism and desire for self-improvement, which limits their chances of success.

In a survey carried out for this study, those who rated their happiness level at 8/10 turned out to be more successful than those who rated it at 9 (*very happy*) or even those who rated it at 10 (*extremely happy*).

The conclusion is that an excessively high degree of satisfaction can fog our vision of reality and our self-help tools can get rusty through lack of use. If everything is already fantastic, there is no need to make any effort at all to improve.

The French novelist Gustave Flaubert went even further, going so far as to state that "to be chronically happy, one must also be absolutely idiotic."

Provocative in nature as that phrase might be, a complete human spirit—and a complex one—certainly needs to embrace both joy and sadness.

As well as teaching us to appreciate life and giving our outlook depth—and wisdom—wabi sabi melancholy has other benefits for our personal life.

- *It is a path to self-knowledge*, since sadness is a mirror that allows us to see into the depths within ourselves which are normally beyond our reach. The melancholic reflection of wabi sabi not only brings us a greater understanding of the world but also allows us to contemplate our own soul—a reflection of what we observe—with greater clarity.

- *It increases our empathy toward others.* Becoming aware of the fleeting and changing nature of life, happiness and pain, allows us to better understand and help people who are suffering, as well as to share moments of celebration with greater passion and awareness.
- *It makes us more artistic.* Delving into the wabi sabi facet of reality brings us new ideas, widens the scope of our sensitivity and feeds our desire to create beauty. It also makes us more sophisticated, to the point of aspiring to converting our life into a work of art, since we know how impermanent it is.

Wabi sabi in the West

Wabi sabi philosophy condenses the Japanese way of understanding life and beauty, but we can find an analogous approach in many places. Examples from two Western poets come immediately to mind—one was Portuguese and the other German.

The early twentieth century linguist, philosopher and poet Fernando Pessoa, expressed his thoughts, feelings and passions through four different alter-egos, or heteronyms: himself, Ricardo Reis, Alberto Caeiro and Alvaro de Campos, who signed the poem "Tabacaria" ("The Tobacconist's").

I'm nothing.
I won't ever be anything.
I can't wish to be anything.
Besides that, I've got in me all the dreams of the world.

We see here the vacuity or emptiness of Zen Buddhism—that it is a blank canvas that includes all possibility.

About the ephemeral nature of life, a beautiful poem was written by Hermann Hesse shortly before he died. The German Nobel laureate had a longtime fascination with the East, with Japanese aesthetics, Zen and the verses of its traditional poets.

In "Creaking of a Broken Branch" ("Knarren Eines Geknickten Astes")Hesse evokes a powerful bare image of the fragility and temporariness of life, but at the same time its heroic resistance to perishing.

Chipped broken branch
dangling year after year,
its cracking sings dryly to the wind,
leafless, bereft of bark,
abraded, yellowed, for a long life,
for a long weary death.
Its stubborn song sounds harsh,
sounds willful, sounds secretly browbeaten.
Still one more summer,
one more winter yet.

A MEDITATION

If perfection is your objective,
it will color all aspects of your life
and you will go blind while getting lost
in the gloomy bamboo forest.
Imperfection should be what you aspire to
in order to see the forest in all its splendor.

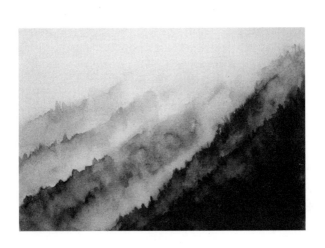

From Inflexibility to Spontaneity

"Relax and be kind,
you don't need to prove anything."
—JACK KEROUAC

A vital lesson of wabi sabi is that things are what they are, not what we would like them to be. In fact, they do not even *exist* in an absolute way; rather, they are constantly changing.

The Buddha warned, as we have seen, that a sure-fire source of human suffering is to wish for that which is by nature transitory to be permanent. Some examples:

- That brand-new car that will soon get its first scratch; in time, it will pick up dents and begin to fall apart. Wishing to keep it like new is to put yourself through an absurd ordeal.
- A friendship that changes with life's different phases. There are high points and moments of medium and low intensity; distance and long silences can form gaps in our understanding. Flexibility is needed for this journey.
- Our body itself grows old and transforms, like shiny iron that exchanges its luster for the rust that lends it another kind of beauty.

What is the sense in rigid thinking or the search for perfection, in a world governed by impermanence?

Let us now travel back in time two and a half millennia, to

the city of Ephesus, where a philosopher of Ancient Greece, who we briefly alluded to in the chapter devoted to Zen was already reflecting on the changing character of all that exists.

We are going to delve a little deeper into its impermanent waters.

The double wheel of change

Just as with pre-Socratic philosophy, only a few fragments of Heraclitus' thinking remain, much of which is in the shape of testimony after his death of people who had heard him speak.

Theophrastus, who directed the Peripatetic school for thirty-six years, said of him that he never managed to finish his works because of his constant melancholy.

Among the maxims that have been passed down to us, we often erroneously cite: *"One cannot enter the same river twice."* In reality, the original preserved fragment says: "*In the same rivers we enter and do not enter, since we are and are not the same.*"

This second translation goes further than the first one, since it has a double meaning:

- The river—life—constantly changes.
- Likewise, the bather—all human beings—changes incessantly.

If everything is constantly changing and humans, in turn, keep on changing, permanency is an impossible dream. We come once more to *panta rei*, "everything flows," and that includes the self.

If we accept that the only certain thing is change—one of the three keys to life, as we saw in the first part of the book —how can we survive without these two constantly moving wheels colliding violently?

Be like water

There are some people whose life is like a classical music score, requiring a particular kind of interpretation, following a pre-determined rhythm, with the exact precise notes. Others are like a jazz jam session, going where inspiration leads them: they play it by ear, depending on what is happening both out there in the world and inside themselves.

The latter would enjoy the river described by Heraclitus, because they themselves are a river and merge with it at each and every moment.

In the mythical final interview held with Bruce Lee in 1971, shortly before his death, this genius of martial arts movies reflects on the absolute value of flexibility:

Don't get set into one form, adapt it and build your own, and let it grow, be like water. Empty your mind, be formless, shapeless—like water. Now you put water in a cup, it becomes the cup; You put water into a bottle it becomes the bottle; You put it in a teapot it becomes the teapot. Now water can flow, or it can crash. Be water, my friend.

Applied to a wabi sabi life, "being like water" implies:
- Breaking down prejudices and preconceived ideas, not making any assumptions.
- Being transparent, without the need to pretend or try to be something we are not.
- Following one's intuition, like a leaf that lets itself be swept along by the river's undercurrents.
- Believing in one's abilities, in the beauty of each and every moment, in the wisdom of life.

- Not fearing life's mishaps, even though at times they may be vexing; trusting in the process more than in the objectives.
- Challenging yourself, doing things you would normally not do.
- Dissolving the ego, merging with what you are doing.

Calligraphy experts drawing the *ensō* circle do so from a stance of absolute spontaneity, letting their body accompany an outline that draws itself. This is the highest graphic expression of flowing with life.

The true path to wisdom

A traditional tale recounts how a pilgrim tirelessly toured the eighty-eight temples of Shikoku in search of the truth. He would meditate and make offerings at each monastery, wearing out his sandals along the way. However, having completed over half the trip, he had found no answer.

Until one day, beneath the golden evening light, he found an old monk under a tree who was trying to capture on canvas the ever-changing brightness streaming through the trees.

He had heard the painter monk described as the wisest person on the island of Shikoku, so he imagined he would have the answers he was searching for.

Without further delay, he sat down beside him and asked him:

"Master, I need you to answer a question that has been tormenting me ever since I began this journey: how can I reach the Truth?"

While continuing to apply small brushstrokes of black ink to his canvas, the monk said to him:

"If you are truly searching for the Truth, there is something you will have to do before anything else."

This answer raised the pilgrim's spirits, who with renewed hope began to say:

"I know! I must practice more, is that not so? Devote more hours to meditating, walk for longer stretches on my pilgrimage, fast and…"

The monk softly shook his head, as his face broke into a smile. He waited for the anxious pilgrim to be quiet before finally saying:

"What you always need to do, above all else, is to recognize that you might be wrong."

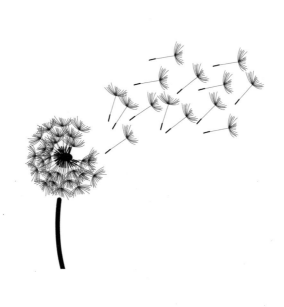

A MEDITATION

I know I have been the same person since I was born,
inside the same body and the same mind.
My thoughts are also always with me,
but if what I think and feel
flows every second of my life…
Am I still me?
And if not, then who am I?

Wabi Sabi and Creativity

*"Learn to cultivate the
trait of humility.
None of us are perfect.
We all make mistakes —
both in our personal lives
and our artistic creations."*
—KATSUSHIKA HOKUSAI

There is a close link between creativity and incompleteness, which is one of the characteristics of wabi sabi philosophy.

It has always been said that the artist tries to compensate for the shortcomings in their own life through their work. So, in some way, the creative act is a challenge to death and decadence—a kind of resurrection.

Franz Kafka, possibly the most relevant Western writer of the twentieth century, had a life that was far from ideal. He had a tortuous relationship with his father and loathed his job as an attorney at an insurance company, although he used the situations he experienced in the courtrooms to write works such as *The Trial*, *The Castle* and *The Metamorphosis*.

In the latter, the most well-known among young people, a shopkeeper awakes transformed into an enormous cockroach. However, rather than dealing with his new condition, he focuses his energies on trying to return to the office that pays the salary that supports his family.

It is a cruel allegory of what the German-speaking Prague writer must have felt when doing his job. However, Kafka found a masterful way of filling the emptiness of what he regarded to be a meaningless life. Each day, on returning home from work, he would take a three or four-hour nap and then write the whole night through until the early hours of the morning.

Thanks to this, he was able to feel complete, even though life is an *ensō* circle that never closes. At death's door, the writer entrusted his friend Max Brod with the destruction of all his manuscripts; thanks to his friend's well-meant betrayal, Kafka's desire to complete an unsatisfactory reality has enlightened millions of readers.

However, it is interesting to see how in Kafka's private life —as shown in his diaries written between 1910 and 1923—the writer experienced solitude:

Being alone has a power over me that never fails. My interior dissolves (for the time being only superficially) and is ready to release what lies deeper. When I am willfully alone, a slight ordering of my interior begins to take place and I need nothing more.

This experience in which the ego fades away resembles deep meditation or even the Hindu Advaita, in which the individual merges with the cosmos until they disappear.

Forget everything. Open the windows. Clear the room. The wind blows through it. You see only its emptiness; you search in every corner and don't find yourself.

A coming together experience

In *The Japanese Way of the Artist,* Sensei H. E. Davey, one of the greatest *shodō* (Japanese paint calligraphy) artists outside Japan and the author of numerous articles and books about Japanese arts, offers some clues as to how wabi sabi defines Japanese art especially well.

"Beauty is not the opposite of ugliness. Rather, beauty lies in a state beyond and includes all opposites; beauty is thus found in naturalness."

Naturalness is one of the wabi sabi principles inspired by nature, where everything is imperfect, incomplete and momentary.

However, as we saw earlier, the creator feels fulfilled and complete when practicing their art, perhaps because, as Davey himself says, *"The present is outside of time."*

This is one of the blessings of the creative act. When a paintbrush touches a canvas, or we place our fingers on the letters of a keyboard, the past becomes remnants of a dream and the future is perceived as an improbable oasis.

Creation is always *now*, since it places us in a state of flow in which the creator merges with what is being created, in an exceptional revelatory experience of togetherness. Japanese arts seek this union of the individual and what he or she is doing, and not just in disciplines like calligraphy, watercolor painting, or poetry.

Just as Davey points out in *The Japanese Way of the Artist,* *"In Japanese swordsmanship, it is not uncommon to speak of a unity of mind, body, and sword."*

Mishima's journey

The works of my countryman Yukio Mishima, who lost out to Kawabata in the Nobel Prize in Literature award in 1968, captured the ability of art and our life experiences to be a means for shaking off what we are, including our past.

This state of flow in which we are "outside of time" is like a journey that takes us beyond ourselves, as is conveyed by this snippet of *Forbidden Colors* by the author who took his own life in 1970—following the *seppuku* ritual—when he was just forty-five years old: *"Undertaking a journey produces a mysterious feeling. One believes oneself to be freed not only of the places left behind but also of the time left behind."*

Undoubtedly, creation offers us this journey. Just as the passionate explorer forgets about the place he comes from, his body and mind exclusively serving the adventure, so is the true artist a tool of transformation.

We too, as spectators of beautiful things—and sad ones, as Kawabata would say—sometimes experience a feeling of loss, because everything that shines is at the same time beginning its deterioration, its star waning.

Mishima explains it like this in his autobiographical work of fiction *Confessions of a Mask*: *"Sonoko's lips glistened and her eyes shone. Her beauty depressed me and made me feel impotent. That very feeling is what made Sonoko seem even more ephemeral to me."*

Passing the magical threshold

Art and a journey—external or internal—as a way of dissolving the ego is in the forefront of Joseph Campbell's most emblematic work, *The Hero with a Thousand Faces*.

In 1949 this American mythologist published his novel idea that there is a common template in the great heroic adventures, even in cultures that have never been in contact. This applies to works of fiction from *The Odyssey* to *Star Wars*, although other authors have added that this same "plot" is to be found in the life history of characters like Moses, the Buddha and Christ.

In Campbell's own words:

A hero ventures forth from the world of common day into a region of supernatural wonder: fabulous forces are there encountered, and a decisive victory is won: the hero comes back from this mysterious adventure with the power to bestow boons on his fellow man.

Among the seventeen common stages of this journey, it is interesting to note how the first ones affect the hero in the same way that they affect an artist just starting out:

1. *The call of adventure.* Hearing of something new, the hero feels driven to abandon the known world and normality for the adventure that is calling them. / The artist feels something new bubbling away inside them, a creative force that demands that they venture into art.

2. *Rejection of the call.* The hero balks at leaving their comfort zone, perhaps out of the sense of duty they feel toward their loved ones or because the new adventure frightens them. / The artist, in their early stages, refuses to believe him or herself capable of beginning their work. They have to fight against their own fears and beliefs before getting the ball rolling.

3. *The mentor or supernatural help.* Someone they know who has greater knowledge than they do, or maybe even a magical assistant, convinces the hero to begin their adventure and gives them their first directions. / The artist either gets the support of a tutor or a flash of divine inspiration. They have no choice but to begin their creative adventure.

In the fourth stage of the monomyth, *the passing of the threshold,* the hero or artist has already thrown themselves into the adventure, leaving behind the known world and entering a new one where they know neither the rules nor their consequences. And then comes the crowning moment, the fifth stage, *the belly of the whale,* in which dissolution and rebirth take place. Campbell says:

The idea that the passage of the magical threshold is a transit into a sphere of rebirth is symbolized in the worldwide womb image of the belly of the whale. The hero (…) is swallowed into the unknown and would appear to have died. (…) Instead of passing outward, beyond the confines of the visible world, the hero goes inward, to be born again. (…) The temple interior, the belly of the whale, and the heavenly land beyond, above, and below the confines of the world, are one and the same. That is why the approaches and entrances to temples are flanked and defended by colossal gargoyles: dragons, lions, devil-slayers with drawn swords, resentful dwarfs, winged bulls. The devotee at the moment of entry into a temple undergoes a metamorphosis. Once inside he may be said to have died to time and returned to the World Womb, the World Navel, the Earthly Paradise.

A wabi sabi diary

There is no need to write a great work like *The Hero with a Thousand Faces* to unlock your creativity and pass the threshold. You can even enter the belly of the whale by releasing your creative energy in the simplest of ways.

Each day write a list of whatever wabi sabi experiences you had. If you already keep a diary, keep on doing so. Simply add a small section at the end of each day. Analyze your day through the three dimensions of wabi sabi we saw at the start of the book.

– *Philosophy dimension*:
• What was the most wabi sabi thing about your day?
• And the least wabi sabi?

– *Art dimension*:
• Which wabi sabi objects, buildings, music or details did you come across during the day?
• What/how did they make you feel?

– *Practice dimension*:
• Did you live by the principles of wabi sabi?
• Did you take time out to do nothing or did you allow yourself to be ruled by haste?
• Did you react especially emotionally to any event?
• To round things off, write a *haiku* before closing the diary.

Exercise: how to write a haiku
1. It must be simple, with three short brushstroke-like lines.
2. It will contain few verbs (sometimes none at all).

3. The haiku should capture an instant, like a photograph.
4. Nature or the urban environment should be present.
5. There may be a reference to the time of year.
6. The artist's feelings must infuse the text.

Close your eyes for a brief moment. Visualize something nice that may have happened to you or that you saw during the day. Open your eyes and write what you visualized without analyzing it or turning it over in your head—just write it.

Haiku examples from my own diary:

springtime blue,
I walk to Yoyogi,
the smell of ramen

businessmen,
walk quickly,
a monk on the corner

a cat visits a museum,
returns to its lair,
purr purr.

snowflakes build up on the veranda,
music by Bach plays,
someone rings the bell

eyes from another universe,
a sakura petal,
the wind leaves it disheveled

silence,
the air fills with piano notes
silence

the smell of coffee,
reading a novel,
end of the story

the sun warms the terrace,
Tama takes a nap,
suddenly a cloud hides the sun

III

Wabi Sabi as a Way of Life

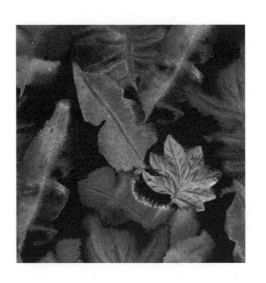

A MEDITATION

the maple tree tinges the fall with ochre hues,
the deer looks up
sketching its yearning in the sky
the twilight clouds watch over us
drawing shadows in the meadows
swept away by the breeze,
while I write

Imperfection as a Road to Excellence

*"There is no excellent beauty that
hath not some strangeness in the
proportion."*
—Francis Bacon

On my last trip to India, I met a woman called Sangeeta. She
is the director of several schools in the north of Kolkata and
explained to me that, on the first day of the new school year,
newly enrolled pupils are always told the following story.

A farmer who lived to the north of Jaipur would go to the
closest spring to his farm every day for water. To carry the water, he rested a long wooden pole on his neck. A bucket hung
from each end of the stick, which he would fill at the spring.

After a while, when he was returning home after fetching
water, he realized that one of the buckets was half empty. Apparently, it had a small crack. The farmer decided to keep on
using the broken bucket for years.

The bucket that always made it back home full was proud
of its achievements. Every day it blamed the other bucket for
the problem caused by its flaws.

"You're always spilling the water on the way back," said the
perfect bucket. "You do half the work I do – you're useless!"

"I'm really sorry… I'm ashamed that the water leaks out
because of this crack I have," the imperfect bucket apologized.

Ashamed of its flaw, the bucket that always made it back half empty began to get depressed and became less and less talkative.

One day, the farmer heard the two buckets' conversation. And he turned to the imperfect bucket saying:

"Have you noticed that beautiful flowers have sprung up on your side of the path, but on the other side there is nothing but earth and stones?"

The perfect bucket, lost for words, looked at the imperfect bucket enviously.

"I planted seeds on your side of the path and every day you watered them when we returned home together," the farmer went on. "Over the last few years, I've been picking some of those flowers to decorate my house. Without you, I would never have been surrounded by such beauty."

The enemy of the good

We can all identify with the broken bucket. Oftentimes we focus all our attention on defects and things that are not going quite so well as we would like them to.

However, as Voltaire said, "*The perfect is the enemy of the good*." If we only see our defects, we will lose confidence in ourselves and lead sad lives like the broken bucket.

The demands of modern life, however, push us to try to be like the perfect bucket. We are expected to achieve success, make money and become popular on social networks, constantly improve following the advice of internet books and gurus....

And that is where the danger lies. If we become obsessed with perfecting our lives, we will end up like the full bucket,

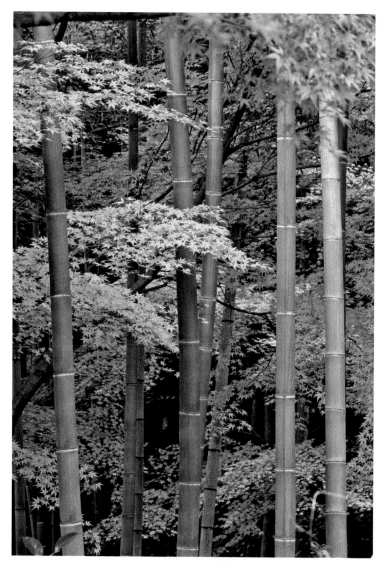

Mono no aware is the Japanese term for an awareness of the transience of things. It is a sense of poignancy, but also of gratitude and joy at having experienced the many moments of fleeting beauty that make up the best part of our lives. Perhaps the life and strength in this green bamboo would mean less without the reminder of impermanence that surrounds it.

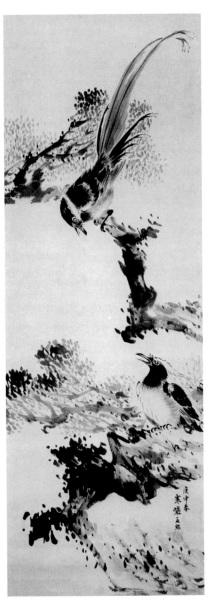

"A Painting of Birds and Flowers" by Kitayama Kangan (1767–1801). *Sumi-e* (which means "black ink painting") generally conveys themes from the natural world. Rather than seeking to replicate a thing's appearance, *sumi-e* uses fluid brushstrokes, varying the brush's pressure accordingly in order to capture the subject's spirit, its essence.

In the arts of *sumi-e* (ink wash painting), and *shodō* (calligraphy), acceptance of imperfection is part of the practice. You cannot go back and bolden a weak line. You cannot go over your painting to correct or disguise imperfections. Rather, you acknowledge the imperfections in your work, and move on.

An example of *shodō* by Musō Soseki 1275–1351, Japanese Zen master, garden designer and poet. The text 別無工夫 can be translated as "no further (spiritual) meaning."

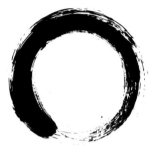

Considered by many to be both *sumi-e* and *shodō*, the *ensō* is a Zen symbol and practice. It is completed in a single stroke, and arises out of the individual in a given moment, It can be wide open or nearly but never quite closed. However many *ensō* an individual can draw over the course of time, no two will be the same.

Closely connected with Zen, *shodō* is an act of meditation. The true art is not in the mastery of a technique, but in learning to empty one's mind, and allowing the letters to flow out of this "no mind" (*mushin*) state. The spiritual (meaning) must take precedence over technique (execution).

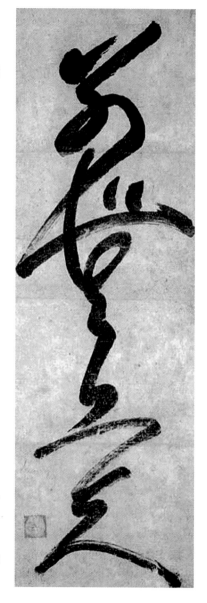

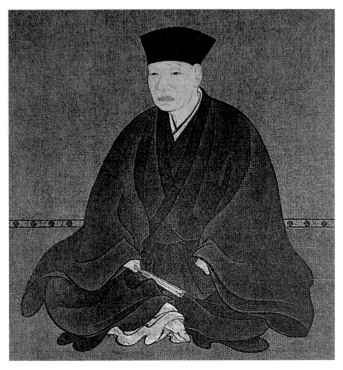

Sen no Rikyū is widely acknowledged as the father of the tea ceremony and also as the father of wabi sabi as it is understood today. In one version of his legend, he traveled in the spring to learn the Way of Tea from the master Takeno Jōō, who tested him by asking him to prepare the garden. Rikyū carefully raked and cleared away debris from every corner and cranny, until the garden was perfect. Then, he reached overhead and shook the limb of a cherry tree, causing a few blossoms to fall on the immaculate ground. To transcend acceptance by actively seeking and embracing what is natural, and therefore imperfect, is one of the threads that make up the almost indescribable thing called wabi sabi.

In poetry, *wabi* might translate as the element in us that recognizes the beauty and profundity in nature—in the world as it is—and *sabi* might refer to the sense of solitude, perhaps of melancholy, that contemplates it. For the haiku master Bashō (opposite page), the aim of poetry is to bring the reader closer to this openness which, in turn, brings us closer to nature.

古池
蛙飛び込む
水の音

*Furu ike ya
kawazu tobikomu
mizu no oto*

Old pond—
frogs jumped in—
water's sound

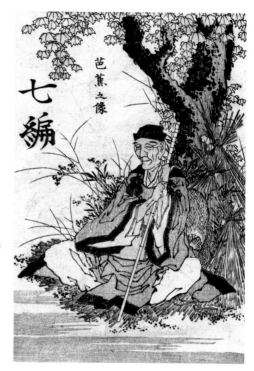

Lafcadio Hearn's rendition of Bashō's famous "Frog Haiku" is one of over thirty translations.

In his *Tsurezuregusa* (*Essays in Idleness*), the fourteenth century monk Yoshida Kenkō wrote, "Are we to look at cherry blossoms only in full bloom, at the moon only when it is cloudless?" All stages and conditions of nature, are beautiful and worthy of our attention, contemplation and affection. Indeed, Kenkō goes on to say, "Branches about to blossom or gardens strewn with faded flowers are worthier of our admiration."

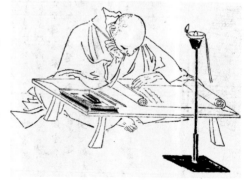

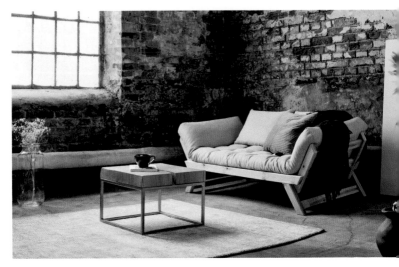

In the West, the spirit of wabi sabi is a trend in planning home interiors, characterized by minimal and simple furniture and working with what already exists—appreciating the beauty in irregularities such as exposed pipes and the wonderful texture and sense of age from flaking masonry, as shown above. Perhaps the most distinguished feature of the wabi sabi home is the absence of clutter. A feature of living in a wabi sabi way is considering how much you really need, not just in your surroundings, but in all aspects of your life. Life is short, and material possessions are only the smallest part of that adventure. Our lives are more fully enjoyed when we travel lighter, and keep our sights on the things that truly matter.

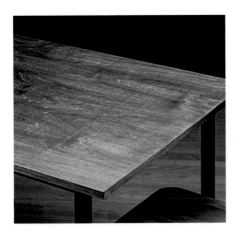

Reusing old things is another characteristic of a wabi sabi home. An old tabletop may be used in the making of a new table. An old sofa may be repaired rather than replaced. A special mug, now chipped or cracked, may continue to be a favorite drinking cup. Using less, owning less, gravitating toward the personal and meaningful rather than toward the latest trends—these are part of a wabi sabi mindset.

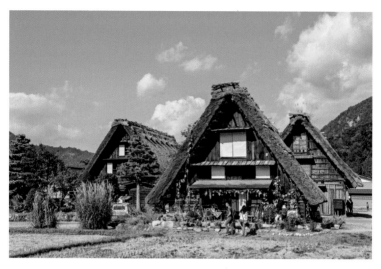

Traditional *minka* houses—homes to the merchant, farmer and craftsman castes before the modern era, were models of rustic efficiency. Although a given house may have a social structure within it, it had no grandeur, such being the prerogative of the samurai class. They were well made, with the materials available to the lesser castes. From this domestic architecture, with its limited space and austere interiors, came the love of minimalism that is still part of the Japanese aesthetic.

The teahouses of the Katsura Imperial Villa are a perfect example of how Zen and the wabi sabi philosophy penetrated even the homes of princes. This teahouse embodies the simplicity and humility that are intrinsic to wabi sabi.

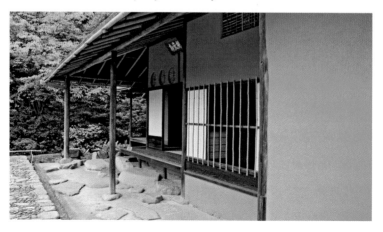

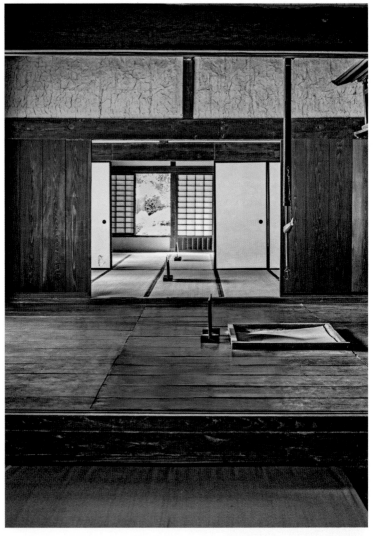

The traditional Japanese interior is almost austere, containing nothing more than is needed. A roof over the head, a comfortable place to sit, eat and sleep, something meaningful to contemplate (like a scroll), something beautiful to look at (like a flower in a vase). The home is built primarily of what nature gives— wood, stone, straw.

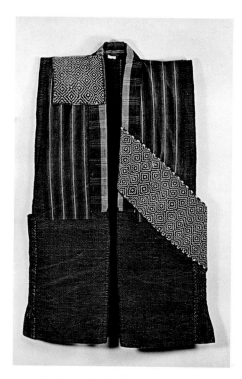

Sashiko is a form of Japanese embroidery born of necessity, designed to reinforce hardworking fabrics or to quilt together multiple layers of worn fabric to make a new layer. On the vest above, sashiko was used to reinforce the portion of the vest that came in direct contact with the band on the sledges used to haul rice.

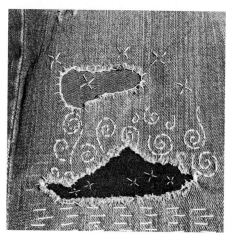

Nowadays, sashiko is used at levels from the simplest to the most intricate, both for decorating fabric and to repair old favorites, like these jeans, adding artistry to the act of restoring rather than replacing. Old things become even more valuable when care, effort and affection have gone into their repair.

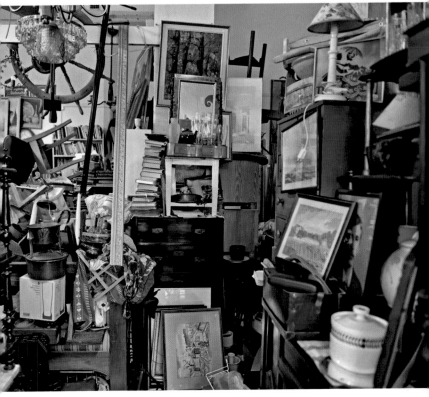

It's hard enough just looking at it, isn't it? And yet the clutter we surround ourselves with in our environment is not unlike the clutter we keep inside our heads and hearts—worry, competitiveness, insecurity, grudges, the list goes on. And yet how much "stuff" do we really need? What is truly valuable to us, and what is weighing us down? We need to clear the clutter, to make space both in our homes and in ourselves, remove all the things we trip over, the things that hide that which is really important from our view. That is a step toward really seeing the beauty around us, and the beauty in ourselves.

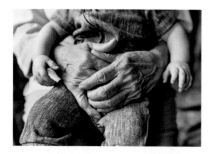

We ourselves are impermanent. The stages of life fly by. We look up, and years have passed, loved ones have passed, and new people are entering our lives. We are happiest when we can let go of what's past, and celebrate the stages of our lives as they come. Each has its beauty, and each has something to teach us.

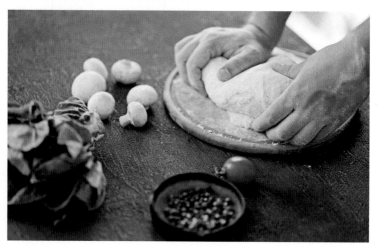

Slow fashion, slow food, mindful eating, mindful everything—"slow" and "mindful" have become everyday buzzwords. And why is this so? In an age that moves quickly and looks for expediency, quite simply, we need reminding. We need to consciously choose to conserve rather than to waste, to replenish ourselves with relish rather than to refuel thoughtlessly with fast food, to be present to the people we are with (even if we are alone with ourselves) rather than pore over the contents of our phones.

The act of mending a garment, preparing a meal—and sitting down to savor it— can be meditative acts. Giving our full attention, putting our entire being into what we are doing in the given moment, slowly brings us back to ourselves. Taking time, restoring ourselves to a state where we are aware and awake to what is around us, is part of wabi sabi.

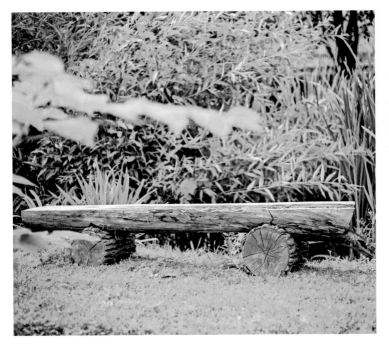

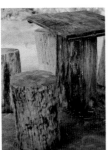 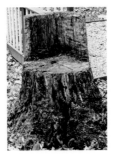 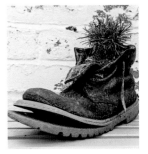

Wabi sabi in the outdoors is reflected in the beautiful collaboration of human ingenuity and the gifts nature has given us to use. A fallen tree becomes a place to sit and relax—sometimes, offering rest right in the spot where it was planted.

When your favorite boots have made their last hike, consider giving those old friends a new purpose.

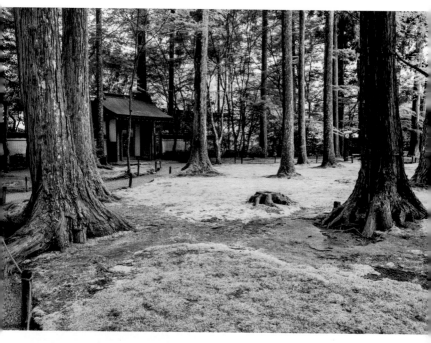

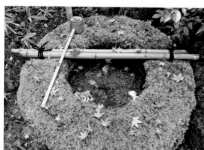

The gate of Sanzen-in Temple in Ohara, Kyoto (above) opens into a world of tranquility consisting of simple buildings and lush gardens. The water basin in its moss garden (left) has been taken over by nature, perpetually covered in soft greenery and regularly serving as a home to leaves in the fall and blossoms in the spring.

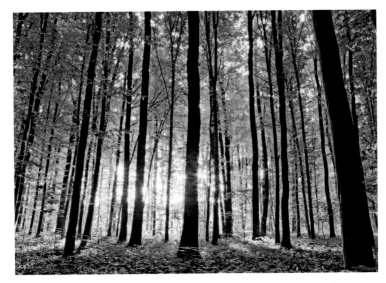

The practice of *shinrin-yoku*—forest bathing—is a wonderful way to reconnect with nature and ourselves. All you need is a forest, at whatever time of year you like best, and silence. Empty your mind, take in the forest atmosphere. Be aware of the stages of life going on, the surfaces of the trees, the scent of the air, the sound of birds and the rustling of leaves in the trees and underfoot. Leave busy thoughts behind. Breathe, and be.

As the great songwriter-poet Leonard Cohen sang, there's a crack in everything; it's how light—and in this case, life—comes through. Imperfection is a gift that often brings us other gifts. Besides learning to appreciate imperfection, we must also take care to notice it, to keep our eyes open and actually see all the beautiful details that are spread before us.

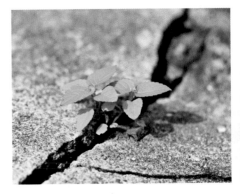

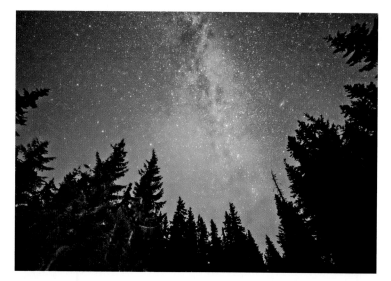

Śūnyatā—"that which is emptiness"—is a vital concept in all contexts of wabi sabi: in art, in the home, in daily life. When we are fully present in the world, in the moment, exactly as they are, we are experiencing *śūnyatā*. When we have filled our surroundings with nothing more or less than is needed, we have achieved *śūnyatā*. When a work of art is at one with its surroundings, contributing to those surroundings rather than standing out or reflecting an artist's ego, that artwork is *śūnyatā*. With *śūnyatā* all things are of equal importance—or lack of importance. It gives us a sense of oneness with all things.

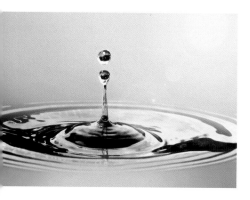

Flux, fluidity, shapelessness, transparency, becoming one with the vessel, moving with the tide—"being like water" is a form of faith and trust in ourselves and in where life is taking us. The fundamental truth *panta rei* (everything flows) applies to all things and all beings. Therefore, we expect our lives and our selves to change. We strive to ensure that we change for the better.

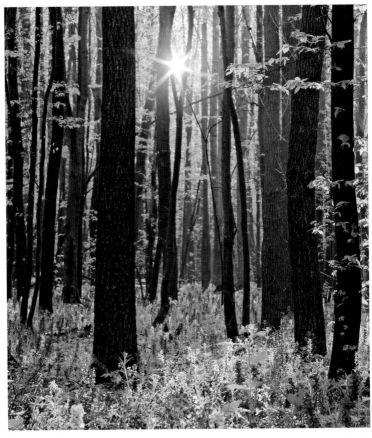

Consider that the sun that's rising through the trees is like no other sunrise that's ever been or ever will be. The sweep of light, the way the colors of the flowers appear, the smell of dew-drenched air—none of these will ever again be as they are in this moment.

The day before you, too, is like no other. The glory of the sunrise is momentary, and the day it heralds will seem to pass almost as quickly. What do you want to do with this moment, with this day?

if we are lucky. Arrogant and heartless, without the space to learn the truly important things of life.

Wisdom is to be found in knowing how to see life like the farmer.

Like the crack in the bucket, each defect is at the same time a virtue, just as we gain something with each loss.

I now propose that you close your eyes to explore inside yourself. Look in your memory for phases of your life when something did not go as planned, but then either something unexpected happened, new opportunities arose, or you learned something valuable that you would otherwise not have learned.

Think of the path that led you to the successes of your life. Was it flat and perfect or did you find it full of potholes, detours and hills?

The best things in life are almost always far from perfect.

A life focused on seeking perfection	A life in accordance with wabi sabi
You never finish any projects because you are always finding little things to be improved.	You learn when it is the right time to finish. Maybe when you feel you have achieved 80% or 90%? The imperfection of our projects—and of life itself—is what spices them up.
You get obsessed with comparing yourself to others. You find yourself in a state of constant frustration because, even if you improve, you will always find someone better than you.	You accept there will always be people who are more successful, more beautiful or luckier than you. Instead of making you feel frustrated or worthless, this is a source of inspiration for you.
You feel you are never enough for the world or for certain people.	You stop thinking that the world or other people expect anything of you.
Obsessed with perfection, you fix your gaze on other people's talents.	You learn to love yourself and to appreciate the beauty and the miracle that is you.
Both your body and mind are in a constant state of stress, because you feel there is always something else to do and to improve.	Given the circumstances, you have done it the best you could. It is time to celebrate and to let your body and mind relax.

You punish yourself with thoughts like: "If I had only done this or the other, everything would have turned out better," "If I had been more assertive, I wouldn't be stuck with this mess now," "If I had negotiated better…," "If I hadn't made this or that decision…"	You know that inevitably things are not always going to turn out well. In life, as in science, we make progress through trial and error.

A long road

Two thousand years ago, Marcus Aurelius was already reminding us that "*The universe is change; our life is what our thoughts make it.*" And there is no rush to achieve this change.

Katsushika Hokusai is a praiseworthy example of this wabi sabi attitude to life and its vicissitudes. A Japanese painter and printmaker of the Edo period, he belonged to the so-called "pictures of the floating world" school and his own life was a never-ending voyage from one identity to another.

In fact, during the course of his career as an artist, he used a plethora of pseudonyms, such as Sori, Kako, Manji, Taito and many more.

Known throughout the world for "The Great Wave off Kanagawa," the first work of his series *Thirty-six Views of Mount Fuji*, the view he had of his art and of his own life could hardly be more wabi sabi:

I have been in love with painting ever since I became conscious of it at the age of six. I drew some pictures I thought fairly good when I was fifty, but really nothing I did before the age of seventy was of any value at all. At seventy-three I have at last caught every aspect of nature—birds, fish, animals, insects, trees, grasses, all. When I am eighty I shall have developed still further, and I will really master the secrets of art at ninety. When I reach a hundred my work will be truly sublime, and my final goal will be attained around the age of one hundred and ten, when every line and dot I draw will be imbued with life.

His beginner's mentality stayed with him until the end. Hokusai never felt like someone who had gotten anywhere, but that as an artist and a man he was a work in progress, like his great wave, which has neither a beginning nor an end.

A MEDITATION

"One step beyond there is darkness,"
goes a popular Japanese saying,
and this contains a great truth which connects all us humans.
We prefer the present to the future because
we have the false sense that, in the here and now,
everything is under control.
The future causes us fear and uncertainty,
because we do not know what it will be like;
it is outside our control.
But the future, at some point,
will become the present.
So in reality, both the present and the future
are outside our control.
And it is beautiful and thrilling that it should be so.

Wabi Sabi and Resilience

"All sorrows can be borne
if you put them into a story."
—BORIS CYRULNIK

One time a piano student asked me:

"Why play the piano if these days my tablet or smartphone can do it automatically better than me?"

He then showed me several apps that played music using scores. I explained to him:

"Your cell phone always plays that Debussy score in exactly the same way. You, on the other hand, with your emotions and flaws, will never play the score the same way twice. You will not play the same way on a sunny day when you have just fallen in love as on a cloudy day when a relative has just died. Music is not just a score—you too are part of the music. Art includes you in the experience; your human imperfections are also part of the work."

In fact, I thought later, when the student had gone, the function of art is not to create something perfect; its mission is to unveil the inner harmony of nature.

Coda: the beauty of the end

Resilience is the art of navigating the streams of life, without letting past traumas condition your present and future. We all suffer life's ups and downs but if we are resilient, we will have the tools to overcome adversity.

On that subject, a couple of years ago a documentary appeared that leaves no one who has seen it unmoved. I am referring to *Coda*, in which my countryman Ryuichi Sakamoto takes a look back at his career while showing the difficulties of his daily life with surprising honesty.

Anyone who has studied music knows that the coda is the final part of a piece, in which the best passages are often repeated. And that is just what Sakamoto does in the documentary, after being diagnosed with a throat cancer. The actor and composer reviews his life, while very bravely and transparently showing us his visits to the doctor, the cocktail of pills he takes every day and the difficulties and uncertainty this life-threatening illness plunges him into.

It is a melancholic and somewhat gloomy documentary, which develops with the customary slowness of old Japanese movies and pays great attention to detail and the nuances of daily life.

As well as this twin exercise of remembering and surviving, there is a third narrative thread that immerses us squarely in the daily practice of wabi sabi. Apart from his artistic facet, Sakamoto is a well-known peace and environmental activist. The documentary shows how, after the Fukushima catastrophe, he devotes himself to a personal gesture that is both remarkable and significant.

After rescuing a piano that the tsunami had left submerged in the sea, Sakamoto tries to restore it with his own hands – an impossible task to fulfill with such a delicate instrument. He knows it is impossible for the Yamaha grand piano to sound in tune again, but even so he tries to rebuild it as best he can.

At the end of the documentary, while he struggles to re-cover and wonders about the future of the world, he ends up recording an album coaxing what seem like the wails of some undersea creature out of its keys.

Sakamoto does not know how long he will end up living, how long his coda will be, but in the meantime saving the wrecked piano is his way of bringing beauty into the world. An imperfect beauty, like the essence of wabi sabi, but in any case one that gives us hope. His message is: not everything is lost; what is broken may be put back together and where there was pain, love and beauty may be created.

There is life in what is broken

Sakamoto's rescued piano will always be imperfect, and the artist will never be able to fulfill his dream of restoring it, because of the extent of the damage and the finite nature of his own life, but even so, beauty remains the heartbeat of his motivation.

From one musician to another: there is an anecdote about Itzhak Perlman told by the writer and speaker Álex Rovira which is specially revealing in that regard.

The following took place when the Israeli violinist was giving a concert at New York's Lincoln Center. Perlman has serious physical impairments affecting his mobility, due to the after-effects of polio, which he caught in his childhood and has restricted him ever since. He has trouble stepping on stage, where he needs to play the violin seated.

That evening, facing a concert hall packed with people waiting to hear his brilliance, having put his crutches to one side and unbuckled the braces supporting his legs and waist, he settled the violin against his chin and just as the orchestra conductor was about to begin the concert, an unfortunate accident occurred—one of the violin strings snapped.

On hearing the sharp crack, the audience imagined the concert would be halted until the string could be replaced. However, to everyone's great surprise, Perlman carried on playing with his customary enthusiasm and devotion, as if nothing was amiss.

In order to play the piece with only three strings, Perlman had to adapt his playing on the spot, managing to give a performance of extraordinary beauty and expressiveness.

When he finished, the audience was left in a stunned silence, and then spectators began to stand up and applaud his achievement, moved by its incredible beauty and resilience. In the end, the entire concert hall burst into a thunderous ovation.

It is said that, after wiping the rivers of sweat from his face with a handkerchief, Perlman bowed gratefully from his chair and then lifted his bow to indicate to the audience that he wished to speak. When the hall had fallen silent once more, the heroic violinist said:

"You know what? ... There are times when the artist's task is to know how much they can manage to do with what they have left."

Álex Rovira reflects on this touching anecdote in this way:

This is the question that perhaps we should start to keep on asking ourselves in our lives: What can we do with what we have, with what we have left? If we consider that we will always lack something, that there will always be room for improvement, that oftentimes we will have to perform our pieces in life with one string missing from our violin... Right there, in this ability to devote ourselves heart and soul to life with what we have now, although we are incomplete and fragile, courage appears: What can we do with what we have left?

The lessons of *kintsugi*

We may answer that question with a Japanese art that is full of human beauty—*kintsugi*, which uses gold lacquer to mend broken pieces. It makes them resilient.

Using this striking golden material, instead of disguising the breakage by using the same color, encapsulates a philosophy that may be applied to the human spirit:

- All objects have a story. By showing their wounds, we allow them to explain it to us and this makes them more valuable. *Lesson 1 of kintsugi: scars are not to be hidden—they are part of our story.*
- If the cup, vase or piece we have mended has had an accident, this makes it more interesting. In fact, this makes it more valuable than an immaculate object that has just come off the production line. *Lesson 2 of kintsugi: what we have survived to get this far is our greatest treasure.*
- The accident that does not make us give up, like Perlman with his violin, becomes a strength and a source of knowledge. As the great Persian poet Rumi said, "*A wound is the entrance by which light penetrates you." Lesson 3 of kintsugi: accidents are enlightening.*

When we have reached a certain age, in one way or another we are all broken vessels which have been mended and continue to harbor life. To a greater or lesser extent, everyone has suffered heartbreak, been let down by friends or relatives, or experienced disasters of varying magnitude professionally or where their health is concerned.

The big question, as the Israeli violinist said, is what to do with what we have left.

In the face of the blows dealt by fate, we can basically take one of two existential stances:

1. Curse our ill luck or blame third parties, shifting responsibility away from ourselves, and do nothing to solve our problems.

2. Engage with our own fate, taking the steps needed to improve the present, mending what has broken so that we may keep moving forward.

This second way is a path that leads us to a profound transformation. After having suffered or failed, if we get back up, we will be better than before, because we will have acquired experience and resilience, which is the art of being reborn despite all of life's accidents.

On this point, the American novelist Ernest Hemingway said: "*The world breaks everyone and afterward many are strong at the broken places.*"

A season ticket to difficulty

A rare example of resilience is the poet and playwright Derek Alton Walcott, a native of Saint Lucia, a small volcanic island in the Caribbean.

His grandparents descended from slaves and his father had been a bohemian watercolor painter who died when he was little. Derek also suffered the death of his twin brother when he was very young, which left a stamp on his memory that would stay with him for the rest of his life.

These dramatic experiences strengthened his interest in art and literature still further, as a healing oil for pain and at the same time serving as a means of exploring and expressing life's difficulties.

After leaving the island of his birth, Walcott would go on to become a professor at Boston University, in the city where he would establish a theater. In 1992, he received the Nobel Prize in Literature.

In his poems there is a strong sense of resilience and *kintsugi*. the art of putting together what is broken. In his Nobel lecture he said:

Break a vase, and the love that reassembles the fragments is stronger than that love which took its symmetry for granted when it was whole. The glue that fits the pieces is the sealing of its original shape.

Like the broken vase, we humans have the capacity to be healed when we are broken, and become not the same, but even better than before. When something is broken, the love we put in reassembling the fragments is more powerful than the love of the artisan who wanted to create a perfect object, or the love we felt for the object when it was new. Love grows better and stronger, not weaker, over time.

There's a Jewish proverb that says that only a broken heart can heal another broken heart, because it knows deeply what suffering means. Because of this, each wound, each crack, makes us wiser, deeper and more sure-footed on the path of life.

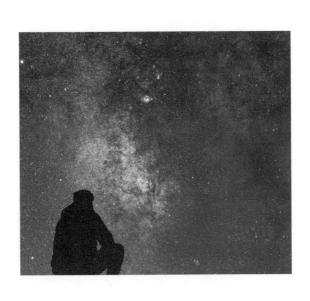

A MEDITATION

I watch the twinkling stars
and look down at my hands.
As I take a deep breath,
a brief pause emerges in eternity.
I am stardust
and at the same time mindfulness.

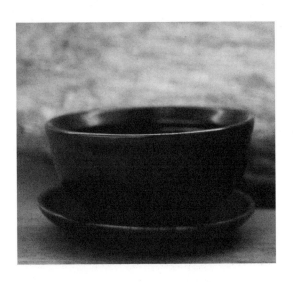

Creating Space

Life is really simple,
but we insist on making it complicated.
—Confucius

Your life is not an email inbox.

We only truly live on the days we have given and received love—the rest is time we shall forget just as we shall be forgotten. When a relative, a friend or acquaintance says to me that they are "very busy," I know they are suffering from stress. When I hear myself answering others by saying, "I'm really busy," I know the time has come to take a time-out and create space in my life.

On that very subject, we have the tale of a Zen master from the Meiji period, called Nanin, who welcomed a university professor who wanted to receive lessons from him. When he arrived, the illustrious visitor took pains to tell him about all his academic merits, his achievements and his views on how the country should be properly governed.

Nanin served his guest a cup of tea, filled it to the brim and then continued to pour.

Seeing that Nanin was spilling the tea onto the tatami, the professor cried out:

"The cup is full—there's no room for any more!"

"Just like this cup," replied Nanin, "you are also full of your opinions and thoughts. I cannot teach you Zen unless you first empty your cup."

Like the university professor, we must empty our lives of everything we do not need and free up space, before adding new knowledge, duties or commitments. That calls for discipline and will force us to change certain habits. It is all about having the right mindset.

What creates space in our life	What fills our life with noise
Setting a limited schedule for checking our email and so on.	Checking our email, text messages and newsfeeds straight after waking up in the morning and just before going to bed.
Deciding on time that we want to spend with the people of our choosing.	Meeting up with just anyone and accepting all the invitations to social engagements we get.
Knowing at all times how to identify what is important and urgent – knowing how to prioritize.	Allowing what is urgent to eat up everything else in our life.
Acting out of self-gratification, rather than trying to please or impress others.	Doing ever more things to impress and please others.
Going for a walk with no firm destination.	Only walking when absolutely necessary to get from A to B.
Doing nothing for a while.	Filling every minute of the day with things to do; if we have a spare moment, we turn our gaze to our smartphone screen.

And it is not just about work or activities. Sometimes, our minds fill up with a constant rerun of worries and unproductive thoughts. If we are really stressed, this can become a crushing weight, and we might be overwhelmed and feel like we're going to explode, like an out-of-control pressure cooker.

At these delicate times, we feel so full that we want to empty ourselves of everything and reboot our lives. Some choose alcohol, drugs and other toxic paths that may feel good for a while. In reality, these strategies are not creating space, though; they are mere escape routes—we always end up right back where we started, at best.

There are healthier ways of creating space in our lives, as we shall now see.

Escapism	Creating harmonious space
Alcohol abuse	Having dinner someplace new with people we love
Drugs	Devoting time to exercise and taking care of our bodies
Out of control gambling and betting	Playing board games with our loved ones
Unchecked watching of movies and series	Planning a home movie night once a week with your family, enjoying each minute that you are watching the movie
Working to excess (*Yes, many people take refuge in work because they do not want to face reality.*)	Only working as much as is necessary, knowing when to stop and enjoying what we are doing
Traveling to escape the stress we feel in our everyday life	Traveling to discover things and to have fun

It's no big deal if we are imperfect

Whenever I am in the Shinjuku neighborhood, I like to call in on the Kinokuniya bookshop. I review the self-help books section, and the general trend I have noticed in almost all of them is that they give us ideas about how to do more and more things to improve our lives.

Most—not all—self-help books give us formulas that add mechanisms to our lives for optimizing our work, being more productive, perfecting our skills and being more successful.

When I read books like these, instead of feeling good, I feel inadequate and I get stressed; it is as though I always have to be doing things, one after the other, to attain excellence. I feel as though these books were shouting at me:

"You have to meditate every day!"

"You have to take exercise every day!"

"You have to do this or that!"

My philosophy is fundamentally opposed to this harassment that many self-help books push on us.

It's no big deal if we are not productive every single minute of the day. It's no big deal if we are not awake eighteen hours a day, pounding away at tasks on a to-do list. We can feel good doing nothing: taking a relaxing stroll with no set destination, sitting down and having a cup of tea while looking out the window...

It's no big deal if we are imperfect.

If we want to achieve happiness and serenity, it is better to set aside things that sap us of energy than to add anything.

The problem is that we are often rushing around so much in life that we do not even know which things are harming us. The first step then, is to start by distinguishing the negative from the positive things in our life.

During my most stressful periods in Tokyo, I used this *Two-Question Diary*, which may be written in less than five minutes a day:

Two-Question Diary

What has given me energy today?
1.
2.
3.
What has sapped me of energy today?
1.
2.
3.

When you have written your two-question diary for one or two weeks, reread all the results and choose three things that were repeated in the "What sapped my energy?" section.

Take action and look for solutions to avoid stepping on those mines in the future. The solution sometimes lies in getting rid of something; other times, it calls for a change in how you approach and conduct your daily routines.

My experience of writing this diary in my most stressful periods is that in the "*What has sapped me of energy?*" part, the same things were repeated day after day. Seeing this gave me insight into the things that were making me feel bad and that I had to start to dispose of.

Ultimately, it allowed me to realize that one of the things that was sapping my life of energy was living in the metropolis, and so I made the decision to move.

Whenever I feel I am too busy or losing control of my life, I use this simple yet effective two-question diary again. It is invaluable for identifying where I can start to empty my cup.

Ten simple ideas for creating space in your life, starting today
I am not a fan of offering formulas, but these ten suggestions are ideas that might help you reduce the strain and noise in your daily life.

1 – Tidy your closet.

2 – Put aside a week in your calendar under the heading: "Personal vacations."

3 – Empty your email in-tray.

4 – Devote two hours on Sunday afternoon to walking alone with your thoughts (Put your cell phone in airplane mode first).

5 – Add nothing new to your to-do list until it is empty.

6 – Write all your New Year resolutions in a way that simplifies your intentions, instead of making life more complicated. For example: instead of "I'm going to go on a diet," write "I'm going to stop eating candies."

7 – Give away the electronic devices and kitchen utensils you have not used for years.

8 – Create an analog corner in your home, or an entire room if you can. When you are resting there, you may only do things that do not require the use of electronic devices. Here you may read, meditate, draw or paint, chat with loved ones, play boardgames...

9 – Free up time on your calendar. Put aside several hours each day or week under the heading: "Personal time." When

this time comes around, devote yourself to doing whatever you most feel like doing.

10 – Breathe in deeply three times, close your eyes and visualize your three best moments of the last week. Give thanks and smile!

Space-creating tool – the wabi sabi cloud

If you feel overwhelmed by all the jobs you have to do, and stress is a faithful companion in your daily life, allow yourself to take a break. Prepare a cup of tea and settle down to writing in your diary or on a blank sheet of paper.

Use this wabi sabi cloud for inspiration. Start the first sentence with one of these words and let your imagination run free to express your worries, hopes and plans for the future.

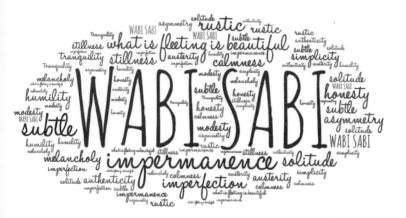

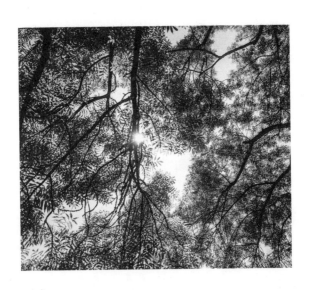

A MEDITATION

to wander through the temple,
to sit down on a bench in the garden
to walk along the beach,
to lean on a rock while contemplating the horizon,
to lie down on the ground,
the starry sky filling your pupils.
the caresses of a loved one,
shared laughs,
a sudden idea

simple pure moments
that cost nothing

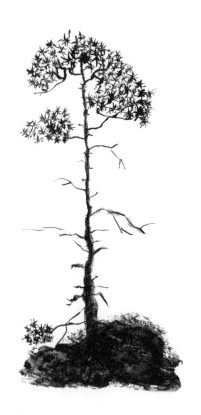

The School of Minimalism

"Simplicity is the ultimate sophistication."
—Leonardo Da Vinci

I let myself be carried away by the temptations of life in the metropolis during the time I spent living in Tokyo. I paid an exorbitantly high rent in Aoyama to live in an apartment just a ten-minute subway ride away from my agent's office.

Each year I would earn more money so I went on a spending spree, buying everything I wanted. I spent several years' savings on a Steinway grand piano (I thought I would play better that way), collected all kind of gadgets for the kitchen (I thought I would do more home cooking that way), started to collect *raku* bowls (I thought that way I would impress my artist friends when they came to visit with me), bought a huge latest generation TV and a leather couch (my friends told me I would impress the girls more that way), bought the latest computer model with a giant screen (that way I would write more and better), and had so many clothes that in the end there was no room for them in my closet…

I was so wrong-headed and confused! Little by little, I realized how crazy it is to collect things that we do not really need. Instead of making me happy, my possessions became a weight on my soul. Everything turned out the opposite to how it was supposed to be.

I felt so intimidated by the Steinway piano that I played less over those years than ever. I hardly had to clean the kitchen because I always ate in restaurants—Tokyo is a food paradise. The only thing I had to do was dust the gadgets I had bought. The giant TV ended up absorbing my free time like some kind of vortex. The computer did not make me write better and having so many clothes in the closet bewildered me in the mornings as I did not know what to choose to wear.

All my purchases were wrong choices made on the basis of two beliefs:

If I have more and newer stuff, everything will be better.

If I have all this, others will value me more.

What have you bought lately led by one of those two beliefs?

When I realized these two spurious mental models were controlling my decisions, I decided to get rid of almost all my possessions, which, ultimately, led to me moving and leaving my Tokyo life behind.

Minimalism time

I soon realized my love for art and wabi sabi had always been showing me the right way. The only thing was, absorbed as I was by the stress of city life, I had ignored it.

Daisetsu T. Suzuki (1871–1966) defined the word *wabi* in the following terms:

Wabi means being satisfied with a small cabin, with two or three tatamis, a plateful of vegetables picked from the nearby fields, and perhaps being able to listen to the spring raindrops pattering on the roof...

Wabi sabi is simplicity and minimalism.

In order to live in harmony with wabi sabi, we must possess only that which is truly essential for us. And to know if something is essential or not, we may ask ourselves these two questions:

1. Is it something I really need and desire with all my heart?
2. Might it be that my ego is what desires it because it feels it will be better at something that way or will please other people?

You do not need to get rid of everything non-essential right away. Start little by little, with as much as you feel comfortable with. Simply ask yourself those two questions on a routine basis and you will start to notice changes in your lifestyle.

Although I confess there is a third question I also ask myself: Is something so beautiful that seeing it every day will make my experience of life more fulfilling?

The architect and designer William Morris said, *"Have nothing in your house that you do not know to be useful or believe to be beautiful."*

As within, so without

There are two reasons why we are reluctant to throw things out:

- You tell yourself it might be useful in the future, that you might be able to make use of it and save money that way.
- It has sentimental value for you—your mind connects it to moments of happiness.

The latter is a very common reason for us tending to hoard things, since this habit usually has an emotional component.

When the hoarding of objects mixes together dangerously with our emotions, that speaks to our mental state. A chaotic room crammed full of objects is an expression of the emotional situation of the person living in it.

Thousands of years ago, the hermit master Hermes Trismegistus said: "*As within, so without.*" But the good news is that if the outer mess is an expression of the inner turmoil, by remedying it we shall be remedying our innermost chaos.

Unclutter your room and you will immediately feel better and be eager to do productive things. You may make a start with these simple measures:

- Throw out ten things you have not used for over a year.
- Choose a corner of your house and make it the most beautiful part of your home.
- Value and be grateful for what you have, without feeling the need to add anything else.

On that very subject, Lao Tzu said:

"*Be content with what you have; rejoice in the way things are. When you realize there is nothing lacking, the whole world belongs to you.*"

A minimalist life can lead you to that state. To help you to achieve it, and if you want to go further than a simple tidy up and want the wabi sabi path to lead your life to a more lighthearted emotional state, you may begin to introduce *danshari* to your life.

Danshari (断捨離): The art of getting rid of the non-essential

This is one of those impossible-to-translate Japanese words. It is written 断捨離 and its three characters mean: *dan* 断 "to reject," *sha* 捨 "to throw" and *ri* 離 "to separate."

Danshari is the philosophy that encourages us to get rid of the possessions we no longer need. Oftentimes, what we hoard becomes an albatross around our necks rather than a source of happiness or security. Because the more we have, the more we have to maintain, protect and take care of.

To adopt *danshari* 断捨離 in our daily life, we may follow the indications given to us by the three characters making up the word:

1) *dan* 断 reject: this is the first step of *danshari* and requires you to choose what you are prepared to reject from your life.

2) *sha* 捨 throw: the second step of *danshari* simply consists of throwing out, or giving away, donating or recycling what you chose in the first step.

3) *ri* 離: separate: this is the third step and is about the metaphorical separation of your emotions from the objects you withdrew from your life.

Danshari does not impose a specific way or technique of getting rid of your things. It allows you the freedom to liberate yourself from what you no longer need at a pace that you find comfortable.

Marie Kondo suggests applying *danshari* abruptly. That is: devote one or two days to getting rid of absolutely everything you do not need. I prefer to take it step by step. One day I sort out a closet, the next a room, and so on.

Whether you follow Marie Kondo's technique or prefer to take it more slowly, the important thing is to introduce *danshari* coherently.

The first step, *dan* 断 reject, is the most difficult to apply. I confess I felt a strong reluctance at first when it came to choosing. One technique that I found useful was to put the things I was not sure if I needed or not in a box labeled "doubting," and if I had not opened it after six months, I could go on to the *sha* 捨 *and ri* 離 steps.

After years of practicing danshari, I feel increasingly strong and free. I am the one who has the power to get rid of anything I want, rather than the objects being the ones who possess me.

I am happier, and contradictory though it may sound, richer.

Living in accordance with wabi sabi does not mean having to get rid of absolutely everything. Keep whatever makes you feel happy and comfortable. Only throw out that which is of no use to you at all.

What is important is to eliminate unnecessary distractions so you may better see the beauty in the landscape of your life.

The American philosopher Henry David Thoreau said that: *"A man is rich in proportion to the number of things which he can afford to let alone."*

Minimalism and simplicity

In order to have a really simple organic life, in accordance with wabi sabi, you need to change your mindset to remove the noise from the world surrounding you.

Modern day society puts more and more pressure on us, offering more products, more new things to learn, more TV series, video games and movies… all of them an arm's length away through the smartphones nestling in our pockets.

Somehow, this way of life always makes us feel inadequate. It compels us to collect more material things as well as more successes. Even if we already have a good job and have finished our degree, we are expected to go on to do MBAs, to land "better" jobs.

Wabi sabi is the opposite of all of that. It means accepting what we are and have now, no more nor less, loving ourselves just as we are.

Wabi sabi encourages us to create empty space in our life instead of adding more and more. In that way, instead of pursuing objectives created artificially by the consumer society, this new empty space will gradually fill up only with what is beautiful and essential, instead of with noise and pressures that cause us stress.

But, how can we avoid surrendering to the rat race, and wanting ever more and better possessions?

For some time, what I have done is to create barriers. Instead of adding more to my life or leaving myself open to temptations, I take steps to protect myself, eliminating what is unnecessary.

If you rid yourself of the mountain of things that you do not need, maybe you will find a diamond in the center.

Barriers to help you achieve digital minimalism
- Create an analog day of the week – for example, Sunday – when you cannot use any digital devices.
- Disable all your smartphone notifications, except those that help you to keep in touch with your loved ones.
- Clear your smartphone of any never-ending applications it may have. What do I mean by "never-ending"? For instance, any social network application in which you can scroll down forever.

Barriers to help you achieve informational minimalism
- Eliminate news bulletins from your life or severely ration

them. Just as we do not wish to eat food that makes us feel ill, so should we be careful with the information we feed our minds.

- Eliminate junk entertainment. Choose wisely the series, movies, and books you feed off. Do not overdo it with video games. What your mind consumes has the power to change you as a person.

Barriers to help you achieve minimalism in your diet

- Instead of feeling caught up in the infinite number of complicated rules a 'modern' diet has, eat a little of everything but in moderation. I follow the principle of *hara hachi bu*, which means when you are eighty percent full, stop eating.
- Practice intermittent fasting. For instance, you may begin by only eating between 10 a.m. and 9 p.m. Outside these hours, nothing. Or if you are feeling brave, you may try with a limited eating window between 12 and 7 p.m., eating nothing at all before or after those times.

Barriers to help you achieve social minimalism

- Eliminate those relationships that are unhealthy. Hang around with people you trust a hundred percent—these are your true friends.
- Be aware that "you are the average of the five people you spend the most time with," as Jim Rohn said. So through your relationships, you decide who you want to be.
- Speak less and listen more carefully to others.

Barriers to help you achieve minimalist exercise

- Choose five exercises to keep fit and repeat them one after

the other for twenty minutes each day. Do not let yourself be confused by complicated routines, with dozens of different positions. The important thing is to be consistent on a daily basis.
–   If you need a more structured program, you may try the Radio Taiso routine (available on YouTube) as used by millions of Japanese to tone their body each morning.

Barriers to help you achieve minimalism in your calendar
–   Set aside one or two weeks on your calendar right now. When those two weeks arrive, enjoy each day deciding freely what to do when you wake up each morning.
–   While waiting for those vacations to arrive, put aside at least one hour a day for yourself, but without establishing specifically what you will devote yourself to during that hour.

Barriers to help you achieve minimalism on trips
–   When the time comes to go on vacation, decide on a place and a date and restrict yourself to booking the ticket for the journey and the accommodation. Leave the rest up to your intuition depending on what you gradually discover in the area you are traveling around.
–   Do not let a travel agency or tour tie you down to an even more stressful schedule than when you are working.

Barriers to help you achieve minimalism with objects
–   Do not buy anything new at all for three months (apart from food, obviously).
–   Devote two days to choosing all the objects in your house

that you have not used for years. Put them in boxes and sell or donate them.
–   Mend the things you like but have not been able to use for a while.

Barriers to help you achieve minimalism in finances
–   Do not allow yourself to be convinced by proposals from banks or other organizations that suggest hard-to-understand financial tools. Decide on a monthly amount you want to save and transfer it to a separate savings account.
–   Limit your minor daily expenses because they have an enormous repercussion on your annual budget.

You do not need to introduce all the barriers I have listed at once—that would be counterproductive as it would cause you stress. Proceed gradually to introduce minimalism to your life.

As soon as you start to use some of these barriers, you will notice great changes. You may adapt them and create your own barriers to minimize the noise in your life.

A MEDITATION

I sit on a rock facing the sea.
The breeze caresses my cheeks
and talks to me in a secret language
that I understand without knowing how.
I breathe and know, finally,
that I need nothing more.

Wabi Sabi Spirituality

"Happiness is your nature.
It is not wrong to desire it.
What is wrong is seeking it outside
when it is inside."
—Sri Ramana Maharshi

Accepting the beauty of what is imperfect in our day-to-day life has repercussions beyond changing our vision of art, creativity or even of our habits.

Understanding the essence of wabi sabi leads us to facing life in another way, both from without and from within. It is a philosophy and a way of understanding life that helps us to dissolve our ego at the same time as giving us a deeper outlook on the world and ourselves.

Embracing this spirituality that beats in nature means a spiritual transformation, the death of what we thought we knew so that we may be reborn in another state of consciousness.

I hope you die soon

It is interesting to see how the modern version of Advaita—the non-dualist branch of Hinduism about the oneness of the human soul and divinity—developed in a city as materialistic as London.

In his book *As It Is*, the British journalist Tony Parsons

explained how he experienced the awakening while on a simple walk:

One day, I was walking across a park in a suburb of London. I noticed as I walked that my mind was totally occupied with expectations about future events that might or might not happen. I apparently made the choice to let go of these projections and simply be with my walking. I noticed that each footstep was totally unique in feel and pressure, and that it was there one moment and gone the next, never to be repeated in the same way ever again.

As all of this was happening, there was a transition from me watching my walking to simply the presence of walking. What happened then is simply beyond description. I can only inadequately say in words that total stillness and presence seemed to descend over everything. All and everything became timeless and I no longer existed. I vanished and there was no longer an experience.

After this experience, Tony Parsons began to promote Saturday evening debates on non-duality in Hampstead, a well-off London neighborhood.

One of the disciples, Richard Sylvester, who suddenly *awoke* in a train station, actually began his spiritual journey after Tony Parsons said something to him in one of those informal meetings, which often began with a walk and ended with them having a drink in a pub.

In Richard Sylvester's own words:

Once upon a time I was a busy seeker, meditating sincerely, being careful with my karma, receiving shaktipat, having my chakras opened and cleansed by blessed gurus, thinking I was going somewhere. Then catastrophe struck. I met Tony Parsons. And that was the end of what I thought had been my life. Tony, who hugged me at the end of one of his meetings, said to me, "I hope you die soon."

Sylvester decided to use that very phrase for the title of his book, in which he explains that spiritual freedom is not a gain, but a loss. Stop thinking you are in control, that you are something distinct from the life that surrounds you:

When it is seen that there is no separation, the sense of vulnerability and fear that attaches to the individual falls away and what left is the wonder of life just happening....There is a sense of ease with whatever is the case and an end to grasping for what might be.

Just as with modern Advaitas, fathoming the profound meaning of wabi sabi allows us to let go of our desire for perfection and control. We forsake any certainty about life, but in contrast to this philosophy of Hindu origin, there is still an observer. An observer that has three reasons for celebration:

1. The daily celebration of the imperfect
We abandon the idea that things should be a certain way. If everything in nature is curved, irregular and bent, so too is the human condition; that means neither complacency nor conformity but love for things *as they are* and development from that starting point.

Thanks to this approach, we may value that...

- Things do not work out the first time around, because that gives us the chance to learn and make progress.
- The beauty that makes us awake to the world is to be found in what is quirky, wrong and unique.
- As well as being a starting point for improvement, loving our own imperfections allows us to love other people's.
- An irregular cup, or even a smashed one, has beautiful stories to tell—just like people with experience.

We are imperfect beings in an imperfect world but if we know how to appreciate the beauty in it, we will find value in every crack or unevenness in life.

2. The daily celebration of the incomplete
We are not incomplete because we are imperfect, but because we are always growing. It is said that no great novelist ever completes their work—they simply abandon it to begin another project that they will not finish either.

The *ensō* circle never closes and we have not come into the world to finish anything, but simply to live.

Thanks to the incompleteness of life we may value that...

- Life is a continuation. If we do not like what we have just experienced, if we feel let down by what we have done, right away we have another chance to do it differently or better.
- The final chapter is never written. In fact, given that life is always an unfinished work, everything is still to be done.
- We come into the world to "pass," but the school of life never closes. Life is a continual apprenticeship and that is what makes it exciting and gives it meaning.

Knowing we are incomplete is a blessing since it makes us humble and at the same time shows us where we may make progress.

3. The daily celebration of the fleeting

We have seen enough deaths to know that we are birds of passage but as Rabindranath Tagore said, *"Perhaps I will not leave any trace of my wings in the air, but I am glad to have flown."* Thanks to the awareness of what is fleeting, we may value that…

- This moment might be our last, so we devote ourselves heart and soul to living it with as much intensity as possible.
- The people accompanying us will not always be there, just as we will not. So we should seize each moment as though it were unique. As the *Ichigo-ichie* adage goes: "None of what we are living will happen again."
- Our time is the most precious thing we have. If, as the marketing law of supply and demand would have it, "scarcity creates value," there is nothing scarcer or more valuable than a minute. If you waste it, you will never be able to get it back.

We are ephemeral, but if we learn to appreciate the moment, that moment can contain all of eternity.

Be the Best Imperfect Person You Can Be

As I write the last page of this inner journey through the beauty of the imperfect, I observe Tama asleep beside the fireplace. I am fascinated by the supreme presence of this cat on the wooden floor. My housemate lives in a never-ending present.

Through the window, the fall trees, which are slowly being stripped bare, make me think of my own existence. Of how fleeting and wonderful life is.

My latest haiku sits on the desk:

I take one step, then another step,
what will I find in the next stretch?
where is the end to be found?

Fortunately, we do not know. The good thing about uncertainty is that everything is possible. Once you accept that you control nothing and that the world changes and evolves following a mysterious script, you stop worrying. And you enjoy the adventure.

Accepting our imperfections is not an excuse for sliding into conformism and standing still. We must take a step forward each day *to be the best imperfect person we can be.*

Here in Japan, earthquakes, tsunamis, typhoons and other natural disasters remind us every so often that nothing is forever. Seeing things through the prism of wabi sabi, knowing everything is fleeting, imperfect and incomplete, will help you to be happy by accepting the vagaries of life, and minimizing the pain when things do not turn out as expected.

You can only be sure of having three things in life: a body, a mind and a limited amount of time on planet Earth. With those ingredients, make the best formula you can for your life, which is unique and yours alone: no one else will be able to savor it—only you!

Dare to be happy amid uncertainty.

If you live your life flexibly following the mysterious rhythm of nature, and with no expectations, the best will always be still to come.

—NOBUO SUZUKI

Bibliography

Ackerman, Diane. *Dawn Light: Dancing with Cranes and Other Ways to Start the Day*, W.W. Norton & Company (2010)

Brown, Brené. *The Gifts of Imperfection*, Hazelden Publishing (2010)

Campbell, Joseph. *The Hero with a Thousand Faces*, New World Library (2008)

Davey, H.E. *The Japanese Way of the Artist*, Michi Publishing (2015)

Kafka, Franz. *The Diaries of Franz Kafka (1910-1923)*, The Schocken Kafka Library (1988)

Kenkō & Chōmei. *Essays in Idleness and Hojoki*, Penguin (2014)

Koren, Leonard. *Wabi Sabi for Artists, Designers, Poets & Philosophers*, Imperfect Publishing (1994)

Miralles, Francesc, *Wabi Sabi*, Alma Books (2017)

Mishima, Yukio, *Confessions of a Mask*, New Directions (1958)

Odin, Steve, *Tragic Beauty in Whitehead and Japanese Aesthetics*, Lexington Books (2016)

Oishi, Shigehiro, Dienar, Ed & Lucas, Richard E. " The Optimum Level of Well-Being: Can People Be Too Happy?" *Perspectives on Psychological Science*, vol. 2, no. 4, December 1, 2007.

Parsons Tony, *As it is*, Inner Directions (2000)

Soetsu Yanagi, *The Unknown Craftsman: A Japanese Insight into Beauty Paperback*, Kodansha International (2013)

Suzuki, D. T. , *Zen and Japanese Culture*, Pantheon (1959)

Sylvester Richard, *I Hope You Die Soon*, Non-Duality (2006)

Tanizaki, Junichiro, *In Praise of Shadows*, Leete's Island Books (1977)

Thoreau, Henry David, *Walden*, Flame Tree (2020)

—*Thoreau on Birds: Notes on New England Birds from the Journals of Henry David Thoreau*, Beacon Press, 1993

Photo Credits

Insert 1

p1 Shutterstock ©Ivan Abramkin/ p2 top: Shutterstock ©Patryk Kosmider, bottom: Shutterstock ©yue734/ p3 top: Shutterstock ©Blazej Lyjak, bottom: from *The Art of the Japanese Garden* ©David Young et al, Tuttle Publishing 2019/ p4 top: Shutterstock ©Patrick Foto, bottom: Shutterstock ©titipongpwl/ p5 from *The Art of the Japanese Garden* ©David Young et al, Tuttle Publishing 2019/ p6 Shutterstock ©Sakarin Sawasdinaka/ p7 Shutterstock ©1000 Words/ p8 "The Great Wave Off Kanagawa" from the series *Thirty-six Views of Mt. Fuji*, c 1829–1832. Katushika Hokusai (1760–1849) Wikimedia Commons/ p9 From "Chiyoda Ōoku Ohanami" ("Chiyoda Great Interior Flower Viewing"), 1894, triptych by Toyohara Chikanobu (1838–1912), from the National Diet Library, Tokyo. Wikimedia Commons/ p10 Detail from "Prince Genji in elegant modern dress in an elegant apartment with the blinds rolled up so he can enjoy the autumnal garden and listen to the cricket's song; a young girl attendant pours him sake." Color woodcut by Kunisada, 1860, from the Wellcome Library, London, UK. Image from Wikimedia Commons, licensed under the Creative Commons Attribution 4.0 International license/ p11 Detail from "Koicha Temae" from the series *A Tea Ceremony Periwinkle*, woodblock print 1897, by Toshikata Mizuno (1866–1908). Wikimedia Commons/ p12 top: Shutterstock ©Pumidol, bottom: Shutterstock ©Julian52000/ p13 Top left: Shutterstock ©SAMoskalenko, top right: Shutterstock ©photoBeard, bottom left: Shutterstock ©Sigur, bottom right: ©PAUL ATKINSON/ p14 top: photo by Fg2. Wikimedia Commons, bottom: Shutterstock ©beibaoke/ p15 top and bottom: Shutterstock © cowardlion/ p16 top: Shutterstock ©geogif, bottom: Shutterstock ©jotapg

Insert 2

p1 photo attributed to Fg2, Wikimedia Commons/ p2 "A Painting of Birds and Flowers" late 1800, by Kitayama Kangan (1767–1801) Itabashi Art Museum, Tokyo. Wikimedia Commons/ p3 left: Shutterstock ©Olga_C, right: Calligraphy by Japanese Zen master and poet Musō Soseki (1275–1351). Wikimedia Commons/ p4 Detail of a Portrait of Sen no Rikyū by Hasegawa Tōhaku (1539–1610) as printed in *A History of Japan* (日本の歴史11天下一統』)1992, Shueisha Publishing Co., Ltd. Wikimedia Commons/ p5 top: Portrait of Basho by Katsushika Hokusai (1760–1849) Wikimedia Commons, bottom: Portrait of Yoshida Kenkō by Kikuchi Yosai (1781–1878) Wikimedia Commons/ p6 top: Dreamstime ©Katarzyna Bialasiewicz, bottom: Shutterstock ©donatas1205/ p7 top: ©Héctor García, bottom: Shutterstock © Sam DCruz/ p8 ©Héctor García/ p9 top: Sleeveless Work Jacket for Sledge Pulling (Sorihiki Sodenashi). Seymour Fund, 1978, Accession #1978.66, Metropolitan Museum of Art, New York, NY, USA, bottom: Shutterstock ©Dixie Grilley/ p10 Shutterstock ©Anna Krivitskaya/ p11 top: Bigstock ©Lysikovaphoto, bottom: Shutterstock ©Flotsam/ p12 top: Shutterstock ©Viktor Prymachenko, bottom left: Shutterstock ©Korawat photo shoot, bottom middle: Shutterstock ©woodsnorthphoto, bottom right: Shutterstock ©Ray Morgan/ p13 top and bottom, from *The Art of the Japanese Garden* ©David Young et al, Tuttle Publishing 2019/ p14 top: Shutterstock ©Ruslan Ivantsov, bottom: Shutterstock ©david n madden/ p15 top: Shutterstock ©Andrey Prokhorov, bottom: Shutterstock ©sl_photo/ p16 Shutterstock ©Kotenko Oleksandr

"Books to Span the East and West"

Tuttle Publishing was founded in 1832 in the small New England town of Rutland, Vermont (USA). Our core values remain as strong today as they were then—to publish best-in-class books which bring people together one page at a time. In 1948, we established a publishing outpost in Japan—and Tuttle is now a leader in publishing English-language books about the arts, languages and cultures of Asia. The world has become a much smaller place today and Asia's economic and cultural influence has grown. Yet the need for meaningful dialogue and information about this diverse region has never been greater. Over the past seven decades, Tuttle has published thousands of books on subjects ranging from martial arts and paper crafts to language learning and literature—and our talented authors, illustrators, designers and photographers have won many prestigious awards. We welcome you to explore the wealth of information available on Asia at www.tuttlepublishing.com.

Published by Tuttle Publishing, an imprint of Periplus Editions (HK) Ltd.

www.tuttlepublishing.com

Library of Congress publication data is in progress.

Published in Spain by Ediciones Obelisco
© 2020 by Nobuo Suzuki

Translation © 2021 by Periplus Editions (HK) Ltd.

Translated from Spanish by Russell Andrew Calvert

Translation rights arranged by Sandra Bruna Agencia Literaria, SL.

ISBN: 978-4-8053-1631-3
ISBN: 978-4-8053-1835-5 (for sale in Japan only)

Printed in Malaysia   2404TO

27 26 25 24   11 10 9 8 7 6

Distributed by

North America, Latin America & Europe
Tuttle Publishing
364 Innovation Drive
North Clarendon, VT 05759-9436 U.S.A.
Tel: (802) 773-8930; Fax: (802) 773-6993
info@tuttlepublishing.com
www.tuttlepublishing.com

Japan
Tuttle Publishing
Yaekari Building 3rd Floor
5-4-12 Osaki Shinagawa-ku
Tokyo 141 0032
Tel: (81) 3 5437-0171
Fax: (81) 3 5437-0755
sales@tuttle.co.jp
www.tuttle.co.jp

Asia Pacific
Berkeley Books Pte. Ltd.
3 Kallang Sector
#04-01, Singapore 349278
Tel: (65) 6741-2178
Fax: (65) 6741-2179
inquiries@periplus.com.sg
www.tuttlepublishing.com